An Atlas of
OSTEOARTHRITIS

An Atlas of
OSTEOARTHRITIS

Kenneth D. Brandt, MD
Professor of Medicine
Head, Rheumatology Division
Indiana University School of Medicine
and
Director, Indiana University Multipurpose Arthritis and
Musculoskeletal Diseases Center
Indianapolis, Indiana, USA

The Parthenon Publishing Group
International Publishers in Medicine, Science & Technology

NEW YORK   LONDON

Library of Congress Cataloging-in-Publication Data

An atlas of osteoarthritis / Kenneth D. Brandt.

    p. : cm. -- (Encyclopedia of visual medicine series)

Includes bibliographical references and index.

ISBN 1-85070-494-5 (alk. paper : hard)

    1. Osteoarthritis -- Atlases. I. Brandt, Kenneth D. II. Series.

[DNLM: 1. Osteoarthritis -- Atlases. WE17 A8806332 2000]

RC931.O67 A855 2000

616.7'223'00222--dc21

                        00-046482

British Library Cataloguing in Publication Data

An atlas of osteoarthritis. - (The encyclopedia of visual medicine
    series)

    1. Osteoarthritis

    I. Brandt, Kenneth D.

    616.7'223

    ISBN 1850704945

Published in the USA by
The Parthenon Publishing Group Inc.
One Blue Hill Plaza
PO Box 1564, Pearl River
New York 10965, USA

Published in the UK and Europe by
The Parthenon Publishing Group Limited
Casterton Hall, Carnforth
Lancs., LA6 2LA, UK

Copyright © 2001 The Parthenon Publishing Group

Printed and bound by T.G. Hostench S.A., Spain

CONTENTS

This Atlas is dedicated to Jill,
David and Susan

PREFACE

In the mid-1960s, when, as an inexperienced Rheumatology trainee in Boston, I presented a new patient with osteoarthritis (OA) to a staff physician, he confirmed the historical features and physical findings I described and then turned to the patient and said: 'You have degenerative joint disease. There's no need to come back here – there's nothing we can do for you. Just take some aspirin for the pain. It goes with aging'.

For years, physicians have considered osteoarthritis a boring chronic disorder for which they had little to offer patients. It has been viewed as an inevitable consequence of aging or a wear-and-tear condition which, once it becomes symptomatic, progresses inevitably and inexorably. Never mind that there is nothing 'degenerative' about the pathology or pathobiology of OA. We have conveyed these misconceptions and oversimplifications to patients by the millions. Apart from the fact that they are scientifically inaccurate, consider the nihilism and pessimism which such remarks engender in a patient.

Today, studies in animal models of OA indicate that the development and progression of this disease may be prevented or, at least, slowed, by pharmacologic or biologic therapies. Clinical trials of disease-modifying OA drugs (DMOADs) have been initiated in humans and prospects for development of therapies that may modify tissue damage in OA are bright. In addition, much better understanding of symptomatic therapy of this disease – both medicinal and nonmedicinal – has emerged within the past few years, so that we are able to treat OA more effectively and more safely today than ever before.

This *Atlas of Osteoarthritis* has been developed principally for the practicing primary care physician, although medical students and residents, clinical rheumatologists, orthopedic surgeons, allied health professionals and basic researchers may also find it a useful resource. Major areas of emphasis include diagnosis, and pitfalls in diagnosis, and treatment. Within the latter areas, drug therapies and nonpharmacologic measures are both covered.

The Atlas provides a focused text supported by clinical photographs (most of which are in color), drawings, radiographs, and a concise list of references. More than mere conceit leads me to assert the relevance of this volume: OA is the most common joint disease and OA of the knee joint, in particular, the major cause of chronic disability among the elderly. In the United States, some 250 000 total knee replacements are performed annually – most of them for OA. The annual number of total hip arthroplasties – most of which are also performed for OA – is only slightly smaller. It has been reckoned that the total cost of OA care in the United States equals 2% of the total gross domestic product of the country!

I would like to express my appreciation to Deborah Jenkins and Kathie Lane for their help in assembling much of the material contained herein and preparation of the manuscript. Both provided invaluable assistance.

Kenneth D. Brandt, MD

SECTION ONE

General information

CHAPTER ONE

The definition of osteoarthritis

In 1994 at a workshop entitled 'New Horizons in Osteoarthritis', sponsored by the American Academy of Orthopaedic Surgeons; the National Institute of Arthritis, Musculoskeletal and Skin Diseases; the National Institute on Aging; the Arthritis Foundation and the Orthopaedic Research and Education Foundation, osteoarthritis (OA) was defined as follows:

'Osteoarthritis is a group of overlapping distinct diseases, which may have different etiologies but with similar biologic, morphologic and clinical outcomes. The disease processes not only affect the articular cartilage, but involve the entire joint, including the subchondral bone, ligaments, capsule, synovial membrane and periarticular muscles. Ultimately, the articular cartilage degenerates with fibrillation, fissures, ulceration and full thickness of the joint surface'

The above definition emphasizes the concept that OA is not a single disease entity. Depending on the absence or presence of an identifiable local or systemic etiologic factor, OA has been classified into idiopathic (or primary) and secondary forms. Table 1 depicts the classification scheme developed in a 1986 international conference on OA.

Table 1 Classification of osteoarthritis

Idiopathic	Bone dysplasias: epiphyseal dysplasia, spondyloepiphyseal dysplasia, osteo-onychochondrodystrophy
Localized	
Hands: Heberden's and Bouchard's nodes (nodal), erosive interphalangeal arthritis (non-nodal), carpal-1st metacarpal joint	*Metabolic*
	Ochronosis (alkaptonuria)
Feet: Hallux valgus, hallux rigidus, contracted toes (hammer/cock-up toes), talonavicular joint	Hemochromatosis
	Wilson's disease
	Gaucher's disease
Knee: (a) Medial compartment	
(b) Lateral compartment	*Endocrine*
(c) Patellofemoral compartment	Acromegaly
Hip: (a) Eccentric (superior)	Hyperparathyroidism
(b) Concentric (axial, medial)	Diabetes mellitus
(c) Diffuse (coxae senilis)	Obesity
Spine: (a) Apophyseal joints	Hypothyroidism
(b) Intervertebral joints (disk)	
(c) Spondylosis (osteophytes)	*Calcium deposition diseases*
(d) Ligamentous (hyperostosis, Forestier's disease, diffuse idiopathic skeletal hyperostosis)	Calcium pyrophosphate dihydrate deposition
	Apatite arthropathy
Other single sites, e.g. glenohumeral, acromioclavicular, tibiotalar, sacroiliac, temporomandibular joint	*Other bone and joint diseases*
	Localized: fracture, avascular necrosis, hyperostosis, infection, gout
Generalized OA includes three or more areas listed above	Diffuse: rheumatoid (inflammatory) arthritis, Paget's disease, osteopetrosis, osteochondritis
Secondary	*Neuropathic (Charcot joint)*
Trauma	
Acute	*Endemic*
Chronic (occupational, sports)	Kashin-Beck
	Mseleni
Congenital or developmental	
Localized diseases: Legg–Calvé–Perthes syndrome, congenital hip dislocation, slipped femoral capital epiphysis	*Miscellaneous*
	Frostbite
Mechanical factors: unequal lower extremity length, valgus/varus deformity, hypermobility syndromes	Caisson disease
	Hemoglobinopathies

Reproduced with permission from Brandt KD, Mankin HJ, Shulman LE. Workshop on etiopathogenesis of osteoarthritis. *J Rheumatol* 1986;13:1126–60

Table 2 Algorithm for classification of osteoarthritis of the knee

Clinical	Clinical, laboratory and radiographic
1 Knee pain for most days of prior month	1 Knee pain for most days of prior month
2 Crepitus on active joint motion	2 Osteophytes at joint margins
3 Morning stiffness ≤ 30 minutes in duration	3 Synovial fluid analysis typical of OA
4 Age ≥ 38 years	4 Age ≥ 40 years
5 Bony enlargement of the knee on examination	5 Morning stiffness of ≤ 30 minutes
	6 Crepitus on active joint motion
Osteoarthritis is present if items 1, 2, 3 and 4 or items 1, 2 and 5 or items 1 and 5 are present. Sensitivity is 89% and specificity is 88%	Osteoarthritis is present if items 1 and 2 or items 1, 3, 5 and 6 or items 1, 4, 5 and 6 are present. Sensitivity is 94% and specificity is 88%

Modified from Altman R, Asch E, Bloch D, *et al.* Development of criteria for the classification and reporting of osteoarthritis. Classification of osteoarthritis of the knee. Diagnostic and Therapeutic Criteria Committee of the American Rheumatism Association. *Arthritis Rheum* 1986;29:1039–49

Table 3 Algorithm for classification of osteoarthritis of the hand

Clinical
1 Hand pain, aching, or stiffness for most days of prior month
2 Hard tissue enlargement of ≥ 2 of 10 selected hand joints*
3 Fewer than 3 swollen metacarpophalangeal joints
4 Hard tissue enlargement of 2 or more distal interphalangeal joints
5 Deformity of 2 or more of 10 selected hand joints
Osteoarthritis is present if items 1, 2, 3, 4 or items 1, 2, 3, 5 are present. Sensitivity is 92% and specificity is 98%

*The ten selected hand joints include the 2nd and 3rd distal interphalangeal joints, 2nd and 3rd proximal interphalangeal joints and 1st carpometacarpal joint of each hand. Modified from Altman R, Alarcon G, Appelrouth D, *et al.* The American College of Rheumatology criteria for the classification and reporting of osteoarthritis of the hand. *Arthritis Rheum* 1990;33:1601–16

Table 4 Algorithm for classification of osteoarthritis of the hip

Clinical, laboratory and radiographic
1 Hip pain for most days of the prior month
2 Femoral and/or acetabular osteophytes on radiograph
3 Erythrocyte sedimentation rate ≤ 20 mm/h
4 Axial joint space narrowing on radiograph
Osteoarthritis is present if items 1 and 2 or items 1, 3, 4 are present. Sensitivity is 91% and specificity is 89%

Modified from Altman R, Alarcon G, Appelrouth D, *et al.* The American College of Rheumatology criteria for the classification and reporting of osteoarthritis of the hip. *Arthritis Rheum* 1991;34:505–14

Idiopathic OA is divided into localized and generalized forms. In the latter OA involves three or more joint groups. For example, a patient with OA localized to the hands but involving one or more distal interphalangeal joints, one or more proximal interphalangeal joints and the thumb base would be classified as having idiopathic generalized OA. As long as it conforms to the above definition, generalized OA may occur with or without hand involvement.

It is difficult to apply definitions such as those cited above to the diagnosis of OA in an individual subject in the community or a patient in a clinic setting. Criteria for case definition in community populations have traditionally relied on the presence of radiographic features of OA. However, the use of radiographic criteria alone to define cases for clinical studies of OA has limitations: although a statistically significant association exists between X-ray changes of OA and reported pain in both the hip and knee, in the individual patient the correlation between the severity of X-ray changes and the severity of symptoms is often poor.

Over the past decade the Subcommittee on OA of the American College of Rheumatology's Diagnostic and Therapeutic Criteria Committee has published classification criteria for OA of the knee, hand and hip (Tables 2–4). In each case the classification schemes are based on combinations of symptoms, physical findings and laboratory and radiographic features. The sensitivity, specificity and accuracy of the classification criteria of OA of the knee, hand and hip approaches or exceeds 90%.

Because the major inclusion parameter in each case is 'joint pain for most days of the prior month', the American College of Rheumatology criteria identify patients with clinical OA. This contrasts with the identification of OA based on X-ray features alone. Because most subjects with radiographic evidence of OA do not have joint pain, estimates of the prevalence of OA will be lower when based on the college's criteria than when based on traditional radiographic criteria.

Bibliography

Altman R, Alarcon G, Appelrouth D, et al. The American College of Rheumatology criteria for the classification and reporting of osteoarthritis of the hand. *Arthritis Rheum* 1990;33:1601–16

Altman R, Alarcon G, Appelrouth D, et al. The American College of Rheumatology criteria for the classification and reporting of osteoarthritis of the hip. *Arthritis Rheum* 1991;34:505–14

Altman R, Asch E, Bloch D, et al. Development of criteria for the classification and reporting of osteoarthritis. Classification of osteoarthritis of the knee. Diagnostic and Therapeutic Criteria Committee of the American Rheumatism Association. *Arthritis Rheum* 1986;29:1039–49

Brandt KD, Mankin HJ, Shulman LE. Workshop on etiopathogenesis of osteoarthritis. *J Rheumatol* 1986;13:1126–60

Keuttner K, Goldberg VM. Introduction. In Keuttner K, Goldberg VM, eds. *Osteoarthritic Disorders*. Rosemont, Ill: American Academy of Orthopaedic Surgeons, 1955:xxi–xxv

CHAPTER TWO

Epidemiology of osteoarthritis

Table 1 Prevalence of osteoarthritis in various populations

Population	Age (years)	Female %	Male %
English	35 and over	70	69
US Caucasians	40 and over	44	43
Alaskan Eskimos	40 and over	24	22
Jamaican (rural)	35 to 64	62	54
Pima Indians	30 and over	74	56
Blackfoot Indians	30 and over	74	61
South African Blacks	35 and over	53	60
Mean of 17 populations	35 and over	60	60

Reproduced with permission from Peyron JG, Altman RD. The epidemiology of osteoarthritis. In Moskowitz RW, Howell DS, Goldberg M, Mankin HJ, eds. *Osteoarthritis: Diagnosis and Medical/Surgical Management.* 2nd edn. Philadelphia, PA: WB Saunders Co, 1992:15–37

Figure 1 Effect of age on the prevalence of arthritis. Reproduced with permission from Loesser RF. The role of aging in the etiopathogenesis and treatment of osteoarthritis. *Rheum Dis Clin North Am* 2000; in press

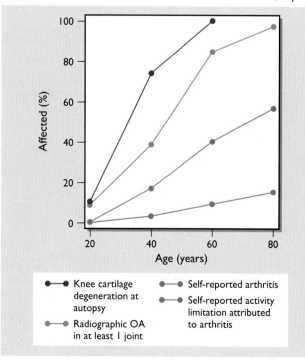

Prevalence

Among all of the specific joint diseases, osteoarthritis (OA) is the most frequent cause of rheumatic complaints (Table 1). More than 80% of all people over the age of 55 have radiographic evidence of OA. Not all of these individuals are symptomatic, but some 10% to 20% of those affected may report limitation of activity due to their arthritis (Figure 1). OA of the knee is the leading cause of chronic disability among the elderly in the United States. However, because of the difficulties associated with diagnosis, estimates of the true prevalence of OA are imprecise; because of the lack of longitudinal data and difficulty in defining the onset of OA, estimates of its incidence are unavailable.

Because age is the most powerful risk factor for OA and the eldest of the 'baby boomers' (in the United States, 76 million individuals born between 1946 and 1964) have just recently begun to pass their 50th birthday, we stand on the brink of an epidemic of this major disabling disease. Figure 2 depicts the anticipated growth of the segment of the population over the age of 65 in the United States, with projections to the middle of this century; it emphasizes the increasing proportion of elderly in the population. Both the prevalence of OA and the proportion of those in whom the disease causes significant limitation of activity will increase (Figure 3).

Risk factors for osteoarthritis

Epidemiologic studies have defined a number of risk factors for OA. In view of the growing frequency of this disease, it is particularly important to recognize those risk factors that are remediable (Table 2).

Figure 2 Growth of the segment of the population in the United States which is age 65 and above between 1900 and 2050. From US Bureau of the Census: Sixty-Five Plus in America, P23-178RV, and Population Projections of the United States by Age, Sex, Race and Hispanic Origin: 1993 to 2050. P25-1104 Census data (1900–90) are as of April 1 and projections (2000–50) are as of July

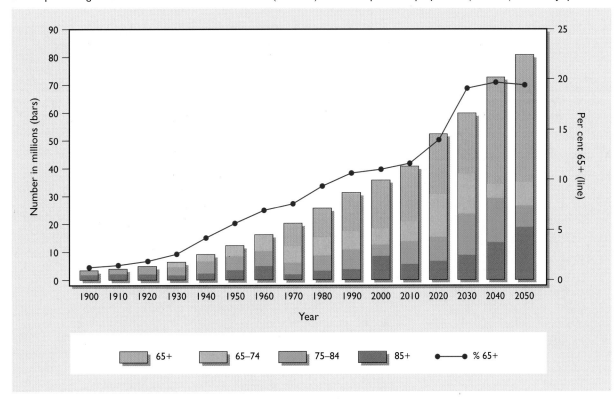

Age, gender, race

Age is the most powerful risk factor for OA. The prevalence of OA at all joint sites increases progressively with age. Radiographic evidence of OA has been found in more than 80% of people age 70 and older (Figure 1).

The National Health and Nutrition Examination Survey (NHANES) found that the prevalence of knee OA increased from <0.1% in people 25 to 34 years old to 10–20% in those 65 to 74 years old. Women were about twice as likely as men to be affected and black women were twice as likely as white women to have knee OA. Others have found an even higher prevalence of knee OA; in the Framingham Study the prevalence was 30% between ages 65 and 74 years and virtually every study that has examined people more than 75 years old has found a prevalence greater than 30% in this subset of the population and more disease among women than men. OA of the hip is somewhat less common than OA of the knee and does not exhibit this female preponderance, suggesting a difference in the etiology of OA at these two sites.

Figure 3 Escalating burden of arthritis in the United States. The projected increases are attributable chiefly to the high prevalence of arthritis in the elderly and the increasing average age of the population. From MM/WA Morbidity Mortality Weekly Report. *Arthritis Prevalence and Activity Limitations* 1994;43:433–8

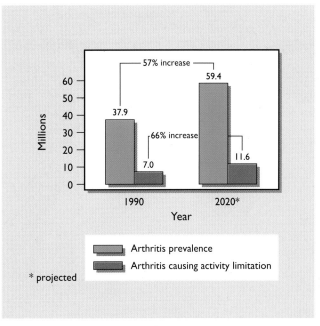

Table 2 Risk factors for osteoarthritis

Age	Female gender
Major joint trauma*	Congenital/developmental defects*
Repetitive stress and joint overload*	Quadriceps weakness (knee OA)
Obesity*	Prior inflammatory joint disease
Race	Metabolic/endocrine disorders
Genetic factors*	Proprioceptive defect*

*Potentially modifiable. Modified from Hochberg M. Epidemiological considerations in the primary prevention of osteoarthritis. *J Rheumatol* 1991;18:1438–40

Table 3 Preventive strategies and potential reduction in incidence of knee and hip osteoarthritis

	Per cent decline in incidence of knee OA	Per cent decline in incidence of hip OA
Elimination of obesity	Men: 27% to 52%	26%
	Women: 28% to 53%	27%
Prevention of knee injury	Men: 25%	
	Women: 14%	
Eliminating jobs requiring knee bending and carrying heavy loads	Men: 15% to 30%	

Reproduced with permission from Felson DT. Preventing knee and hip osteoarthritis. *Bull Rheum Dis* 1998;47:1–8

Figure 4 Trimalleolar fracture of the ankle (antero-posterior view). The fracture in this patient is intra-articular and the tibiotalar joint is displaced. This injury almost invariably leads to OA of the ankle

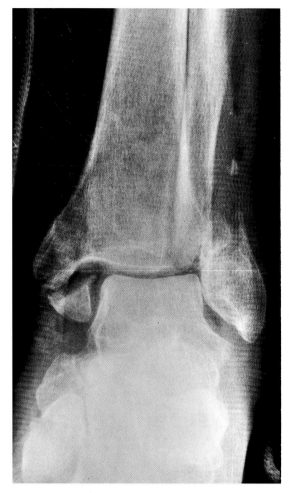

Figure 5 Femoral condyles of a dog which had undergone unilateral anterior cruciate ligament transection 3 months earlier. This is a widely employed animal model of OA and eventually leads to full-thickness loss of articular cartilage on the weight-bearing surfaces of the unstable knee. Prominent osteophytes have already developed in the OA knee, but only mild roughening of the cartilage surface is present at this stage. Note the normal contours of the condyle and trochlea of the contralateral knee (left); scale in cm

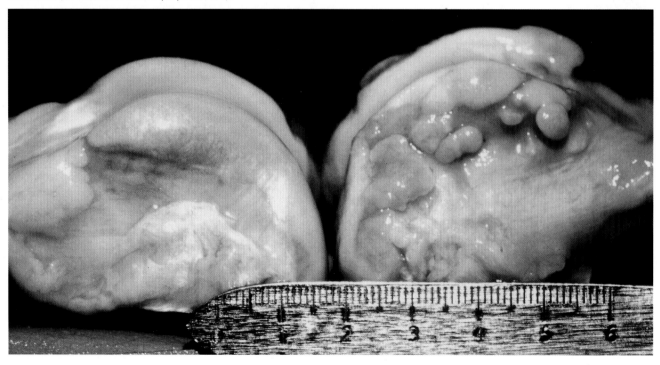

Trauma, repetitive stress

Major trauma and repetitive stress have both been implicated as causes of OA. For example, the patient with a trimalleolar fracture (Figure 4) will almost certainly develop ankle OA. Studies of humans and animal models demonstrate that a loss of anterior cruciate ligament integrity (Figure 5), damage to the meniscus, and meniscectomy lead to knee OA. Even if the cartilage is not involved at the time of joint injury, it will degenerate rapidly if the joint is unstable. It has been suggested that prevention of knee injury would decrease the incidence of knee OA in men by some 25% and in women by nearly 15% (Table 3).

The pattern of joint involvement in OA is influenced by prior vocational or avocational overload. For example, case–control studies have shown that activities performed by jackhammer operators, shipyard workers, coal miners and others lead to OA in the joint(s) exposed to repetitive occupational use. Occupational overuse of the knee joint in jobs which require repeated kneeling or squatting or bending and lifting of heavy loads is a risk factor for knee OA. It has been calculated that elimination of such jobs would decrease the incidence of knee OA in men by 15–30% (Table 3). Farming carries an especially high risk of hip OA, although the basis for this association has not been elucidated. The effect of physical activity as a determinant of knee OA may be stronger among obese individuals.

If major trauma is excluded, the association between specific athletic activities, especially leisure time rather than professional activities, and OA is somewhat tenuous. In the absence of knee injury, long distance running and jogging as recreational activities do not appear to increase the risk for development of knee OA. Thus, repetitive joint usage of the type associated with athletics – even long-distance running – does not appear to cause the joint degeneration which is seen with repetitive occupational use, as in jackhammer operators, shipyard workers, coal miners and others, and may be due to the lack of good long-term studies and the difficulties associated with the retrospective assessment of activities. Selection bias (i.e. early discontinuation of the athletic activity by those with damaged joints) may account for the discrepancy, although it may also be due to the intensity and

Table 4 Body weight and histological scores in 18-month-old diet-restricted and *ad libitum*-fed male guinea pigs

	Diet-restricted (n = 9)	Ad libitum-fed (n = 9)
Body weight (g)	919 ± 21*	1296 ± 44
Tibial cartilage degeneration score	8.00 ± 0.48	11.50 ± 0.47
Tibial osteophyte score	1.33 ± 0.21	2.69 ± 0.12
Femoral cartilage degeneration score	1.56 ± 0.63	9.81 ± 0.63
Femoral osteophyte score	0.00 ± 0.00	0.13 ± 0.13
Synovial score	0.78 ± 0.15*	2.63 ± 0.22
Total joint score	11.67 ± 1.12*	26.75 ± 1.20
Total animal score	23.33 ± 2.93*	53.50 ± 2.92

*$p \leq 0.001$ vs. *ad libitum*-fed controls, by Dunnett's 2-tailed *t*-test. Reproduced with permission from Bendele AM, Hulman JF. Effects of body weight restriction on the development and progression of spontaneous osteoarthritis in guinea pigs. *Arthritis Rheum* 1991;34:1180–4

Table 5 Peak torque in knee extension (quadriceps strength), in ft–lbs, adjusted for body weight

	OA*, pain	OA*, no pain	No OA, no pain
Women			
Number of subjects	35	35	132
Age (years)	71.5	71.2	70.9
Peak torque, 60°/sec	0.40 ± 0.20	0.45 ± 0.18	0.59 ± 0.20
Peak torque, 120°/sec	0.28 ± 0.13	0.29 ± 0.13	0.38 ± 0.16
Men			
Number of subjects	24	33	135
Age (years)	72.2	72.4	71.5
Peak torque, 60°/sec	0.48 ± 0.16	0.59 ± 0.17	0.65 ± 0.20
Peak torque, 120°/sec	0.35 ± 0.13	0.43 ± 0.17	0.49 ± 0.19

*OA = Kellgren & Lawrence grade ≥2. Quadriceps strength of 35 women and 33 men with knee pain but no radiographic changes of OA was not significantly different from that of normal age- and sex-matched controls (i.e., 'no OA, no pain' group). In this cross-sectional analysis, quadriceps strength of women with X-ray changes of OA but no history of knee pain was not significantly different from that of women with OA who had knee pain, and was markedly lower than that of the controls

Table 6   Relationship of muscle mass in the lower extremity to body weight in elderly women with and without radiographic changes of osteoarthritis

Categorization	Number of subjects	Number of knees	Body weight kg ± SD	Lower extremity muscle mass kg ± SE	Correlation between lower extremity muscle mass and body weight	
					r	p
Radiographically normal	107	214	66.13 ± 10.7	6.28 ± 0.07	0.595	0.001
Unilateral OA	21	21	77.14 ± 15.88*	6.86 ± 0.18**	0.850	0.001

Not only exercise, but also obesity is a cause of increased quadriceps muscle bulk. The increase in muscle mass is needed to support the extra adipose load. Muscle mass was determined by dual X-ray absorptiometry (DXA). In comparison with subjects whose knee X-rays were normal: *p < 0.001; **p = 0.002

duration of the activity. Occupational use usually involves repeated exposure over many hours of the day, while exposure of the joint to injury by athletes occurs much less frequently. On the other hand, elite athletes (e.g., soccer players, runners, football players) who participate in sports at a highly competitive level, or athletes who have incurred joint injuries, appear to have an increased risk of developing OA, in comparison with people who participate in low impact sports. A study of former elite long-distance runners and tennis players found a 2–3-fold increase in the risk of radiographic OA in knees and hips. In another study, the prevalence of radiographic evidence of knee OA was 4.2% in non-elite former soccer players and 15.5% in elite former players but only 1.6% in controls. Furthermore, the effects of high-impact loading of the knee and injury as risk factors for knee OA may be independent; in a study of 77 soccer players

20–30 years after knee-joint injuries and partial meniscectomy, 25% of those with an intact anterior cruciate ligament, but 71% of those who had ruptured the ligament, had knee OA.

Obesity

Increased body mass is associated with a marked increase in the prevalence of knee OA. This striking association with obesity is much less apparent for hip OA. The Framingham data show that being overweight as a young adult – long before any symptoms of OA had developed – strongly predicted the appearance of knee OA in a 36-year period to follow-up. For those in the highest quintile for body mass index at the baseline examination, the relative risk for developing knee OA during this interval was 1.5 for men and 2.1 for women. For severe OA, the relative risk rose to 1.9 for men and 3.2 for women, suggesting that obesity plays an even greater role in

Table 7   Progression of X-ray changes of knee osteoarthritis in relation to baseline quadriceps strength

Sex	OA at follow-up	Knees (n)	Peak extensor torque at 60°/sec, lb–ft	
			Per kg body weight	Per lower extremity lean tissue mass
Female	–	175	0.57 ± 0.20	0.60 ± 0.20
Female	+	11	0.45 ± 0.26*	0.48 ± 0.24*
Male	–	205	0.65 ± 0.22	0.56 ± 0.16
Male	+	15	0.60 ± 0.21	0.55 ± 0.21

Among women with no X-ray changes of OA at baseline who developed knee OA at follow-up examination some 2.5 years later, mean quadriceps strength, measured as peak extensor torque, was significantly lower at baseline than that in women who did not develop OA. This suggests that quadriceps weakness is a risk factor for knee OA

Figure 6 Dideoxynucleotide sequencing of normal and mutant alleles from unaffected and affected members of the family depicted in Figure 7. The affected region of exon 31 is depicted; an asterisk marks the single base mutation that converts the codon CGT for arginine at position 519 of the α1 (II) chain to TGT for cysteine. From Ala-Kokko L, Baldwin CT, Moskowitz RW, *et al.* Single base mutation in type II procollagen gene (COL2A1) as a cause of primary osteoarthritis associated with a mild chondrodysplasia. *Proc Natl Acad Sci USA* 1990;87:6565–8

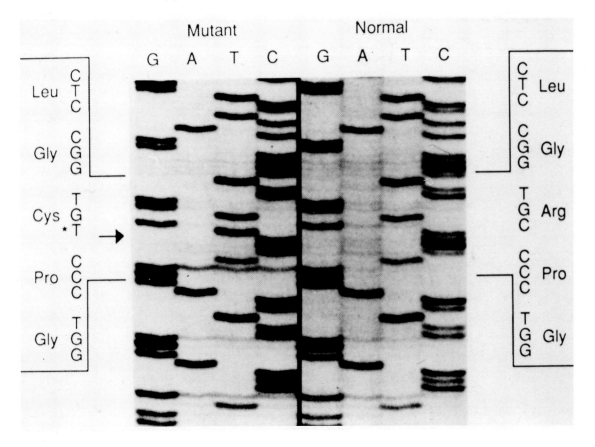

Figure 7 Pedigree of kindred with generalized OA and mild chondrodysplasia associated with a mutation at positions 519 of the α1(II) chain, resulting in conversion of the codon CGT for arginine to TGT for cysteine. Purple squares and circles depict affected males and females, respectively. Slashes denote deceased family members. Reproduced with permission from Knowlton RG, Katzenstein PL, Moskowitz RW, *et al.* Genetic linkage of a polymorphism in the type II procollagen gene (COL2A1) to primary osteoarthritis associated with mild chondrodysplasia. *N Engl J Med* 1990;322:526–30

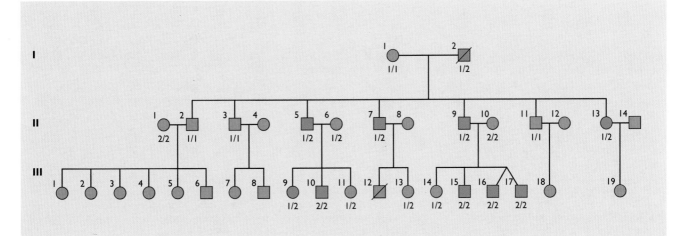

Table 8 Odds ratio obtained from predicting prevalent radiographic and prevalent symptomatic tibiofemoral osteoarthritis

Independent variable	Odds ratio (95% CI)	
	Radiographic OA	**Symptomatic OA**
Sex (female compared with male)	1.58 (0.96–2.59)	1.37 (0.71–2.63)
Weight (per 5 kg)	1.05 (1.03–1.07)	1.05 (1.03–1.06)
Age (per 5 years)	1.38 (1.12–1.72)	1.42 (1.07–1.85)
Knee-extensor strength (per 10 lb–ft)	0.80 (0.71–0.90)	0.71 (0.59–0.87)

Modified from Slemenda C, Brandt KD, Heilman MS, *et al.* Quadriceps weakness and osteoarthritis of the knee. *Ann Intern Med* 1997;127:97–104

Table 9 Relationship between leg strength and rate of loading during gait in females. Comparison of sedentary subjects with those who participated in an aerobic conditioning program and subjects who participated in a strength training program

	Sedentary	Aerobic training	Strength training
Number of subjects	18	19	19
Weight, kg	78.25 ± 3.68	60.53 ± 1.83*	63.06 ± 2.46*
Quadriceps strength, concentric[†]	1.68 ± 0.07	2.02 ± 0.07*	2.10 ± 0.08*
Quadriceps strength, eccentric[†]	2.63 ± 0.10	3.49 ± 0.18*	3.50 ± 0.14*
Hamstring strength, concentric[†]	0.91 ± 0.04	1.07 ± 0.05*	1.08 ± 0.04*
Hamstring strength, eccentric[†]	1.34 ± 0.08	1.59 ± 0.08	1.60 ± 0.07*
Rate of loading of the knee (% wt/ms)	2.21 ± 0.15	2.14 ± 0.15	1.82 ± 0.10*

*Significantly different from the sedentary group; [†]Nm/kg. Reproduced from Meyer A, Thompson KR, Mikesky AE. The relationship between leg strength and rate of loading during gait in females. *J Strength Cond Res* 1997;11:284

Table 10 Radiographic abnormalities in members of a family with primary osteoarthritis and mild chondrodysplasia*

Family member (age)	Spine	MCP	Hips	Knees	Shoulders	Elbows	Wrists	PIP	DIP
I–2[†]	S, OA	–	OA	–	OA	–	–	–	–
II–5 (49)	S, OA	OA, F	OA	OA	OA	OA	OA	OA	OA, H
II–7 (47)[‡]	S, OA	OA, F	OA	OA	OA	–	OA	OA	OA, H
II–9 (43)[‡]	S, OA	OA, F	OA	OA	OA	OA	OA	OA	OA, H
II–13 (38)	S, OA	OA, F	OA	–	–	–	OA	OA	OA
III–9 (28)	S, OA	OA	OA	–	–	N	N	N	N
III–10 (16)	S	OA	OA	–	–	OD	N	N	N
III–15 (17)	S	N	N	N	N	–	N	N	N
III–16 (15)	S	N	N	N	N	–	N	N	N
III–17 (15)	S	N	N	N	N	–	N	N	N

*MCP, metacarpophalangeal joints; PIP, proximal interphalangeal joints; DIP, distal interphalangeal joints; S, spinal changes of both thoracic and lumbar regions with irregular end plates, Schnorl's nodes, flattening of the vertebrae, and wedge-shaped deformities; OA, osteoarthritis; F, flattening of the metacarpal heads; H, Heberden's nodes; N, normal; OD, bilateral osteochondritis dissecans of the capitellum. [†]Died at the age of 75; [‡]osteoarthritis of the ankles and metatarsophalangeal joints was also present. Reproduced with permission from Knowlton RG, Katzenstein PL, Moskowitz RW, *et al.* Genetic linkage of a polymorphism in the type II procollagen gene (COL2A1) to primary osteoarthritis associated with mild chondrodysplasia. *N Engl J Med* 1990;322:526–30

the etiology of the most serious cases of knee OA. It has been estimated that elimination of obesity would decrease the incidence of knee OA by approximately 25–50%, and of hip OA by as much as 25% or more (Table 3). In guinea pigs which were genetically predisposed to develop OA as they age and gain weight, dietary restriction resulting in a decrease in weight of approximately 30%, relative to controls which were fed *ad libitum*, resulted in a decrease of more than 50% in the total joint pathology score (Table 4). It appears that obese human subjects who have not yet developed OA can reduce their risk by losing weight: in women of average height a weight loss of only 5 kg was associated with a 50% reduction in the odds of developing symptomatic knee OA.

Periarticular muscle weakness

It is well recognized that quadriceps muscle weakness is common in patients with knee OA, in whom it has generally been ascribed to disuse atrophy, which is presumed to develop because the patient minimizes usage of the painful limb. However, quadriceps weakness may exist also in subjects with knee OA who have no history of joint pain and in whom the bulk of the quadriceps muscle is not diminished, but is normal or even increased (Table 5) as a result of their obesity (Table 6). Longitudinal studies suggest that quadriceps weakness may not only result from painful knee OA, but may itself be a risk factor for the development of structural damage to the knee. Among women with no radiographic evidence of knee OA at the initial examination but who had definite OA changes on X-rays obtained, on average, 30 months later, baseline knee extensor strength was significantly lower ($p < 0.04$), whether adjusted for body weight or in the lower extremity muscle mass, than that in women who did not develop X-ray changes of OA (Table 7).

When the presence of knee OA (based on X-ray changes, with or without knee pain) as a function of sex, body weight, age and lower-extremity strength was modeled, it was found that each 10-lb–ft increase in knee extensor strength was associated with a 20% reduction in the odds of developing radiographic OA and a 29% reduction in the odds of developing symptomatic knee OA. A relatively small increase in strength (approximately 20% of the

Figure 8 Normal bone (a) and severely osteoporotic bone due to estrogen deficiency (b). Note the thinning of the bony struts, multiple breaks (microfactures), and discontinuity of the normal 3-dimensional lattice which is necessary for strength of the bone. While osteoporosis is a risk factor for fracture, it may protect against development of OA. Reproduced from Kinney JH, et al. Three-dimensional microscopy of trabecular bone. *J Bone Miner Res* 1995;10:267–70, with permission of the American Society for Bone and Mineral Research

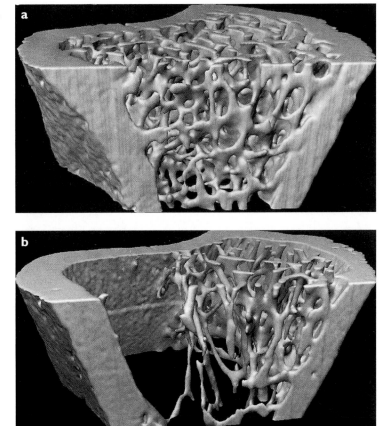

Table 11 Factors associated with progression of knee osteoarthritis

| Older age |
| Female sex |
| Overweight |
| Heberden's nodes |
| Low dietary intake of vitamin C (?) |
| Low dietary intake of vitamin D (?) |

Figure 9 Radiograph of the pelvis of a patient with osteopetrosis, showing the exceedingly dense bone. Patients with this condition who survive to adulthood typically develop severe generalized OA

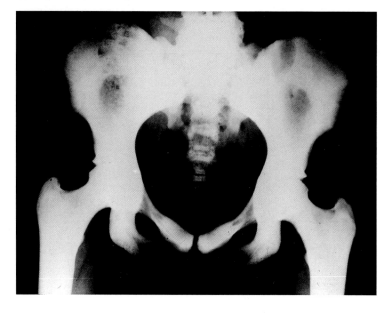

mean for men and 25% for women) was predicted to result in a 20–30% decrease in the odds of having knee OA (Table 8).

The importance of the quadriceps muscle in protecting against mechanical damage to the knee lies in the fact that it is the major anti-gravity muscle of the lower extremity and serves as a brake on the pendular action of the lower limb during ambulation, minimizing the forces generated with heelstrike (Table 9). In addition, the quadriceps is important in stabilizing the knee joint. Hence, weakness may generate abnormal stresses on the joint. A placebo-controlled exercise trial is currently in progress to determine whether strengthening of the quadriceps muscle can prevent development of knee pain and joint damage in elderly individuals.

Genetic factors

The mother of a woman with distal interphalangeal joint OA (Heberden's nodes) is twice as likely to exhibit nodal OA – and the proband's sister three times as likely – as the mother and sister of a non-affected woman. The mechanism appears to involve autosomal dominant transmission in females and recessive inheritance in men. The overall prevalence of Heberden's nodes is 10 times greater in women than in men.

In 1990 a point mutation was identified in the cDNA coding for type II collagen, resulting in a switch from arginine to cysteine at position 519 in the fibrillar α (II) chain (Figure 6). This abnormality was shown to be associated with familial chondro-dysplasia and polyarticular secondary OA in several generations of a kindred (Figure 7). This provided a clear example of OA developing in association with a generalized genetic defect in the matrix of arti-cular cartilage. Transcription defects resulting in single amino acid substitutions at other sites on the type II collagen molecule have subsequently been detected in individuals from additional kindreds with a heritable form of OA, although studies of phenotypically similar kindreds have not revealed any evidence of a mutation. It is possible, however, that defects also exist, for example, in the proteo-glycan core protein, minor collagens or noncollage-nous protein, or in enzymes responsible for the biosynthesis of key matrix macromolecules, but have not yet been identified.

For example, defects in type IX and type XI collagen have been associated with OA changes in animal models. Transgenic mice which expressed α1(IX) collagen chains with a central deletion were shown to develop OA changes in association with mild chondrodysplasia. Other investigators have shown that mice which were deficient in α1(IX) collagen developed severe OA. Genetic abnormali-ties in type XI collagen, another one of the minor cartilage collagens of articular cartilage, have also been associated with OA and underlying spondy-loepiphyseal dysplasia in humans.

Pseudoachondroplasia and multiple epiphy-seal dysplasia, both of which are chondrodysplasias, are characterized by short stature and early-onset OA. Genes for both of these disorders have been localized to the short arm of chromosome 19, to which the gene for cartilage oligomeric matrix protein (COMP), a noncollagenous protein synthe-sized by chondrocytes, has also been localized. Mutations in COMP have been identified recently in patients with these disorders.

Local stresses related to joint use and the degree of deformity due to the chondrodysplasia presumably influenced the appearance of OA in some joints, but not others, in affected members of the above kindreds. It should be emphasized, how-ever, that in those cases of OA in which a genetic defect has been identified, the clinical picture is

Table 12 Percentage of the US population that recalled having at least one month of daily knee pain in the past year, compared with prevalence of radiographic arthritis*

Age (years)	Men		Women	
	Knee pain (%)	Radiographic arthritis (%)	Knee pain (%)	Radiographic arthritis (%)
23–34	5.7	NA	5.2	NA
35–44	7.4	NA	8.1	NA
45–54	12	2.3	11.5	3.6
55–64	11.5	4	15	7.2
65–74	14.9	8.4	19.7	17.9
25–74	9.5	NA	10.9	NA

*Data are from the National Center for Health Statistics. NA, not available. Modified from Hadler N. Why does the patient with osteoarthritis hurt? In Brandt KD, Doherty M, Lohmander SL, eds. *Textbook of Osteoarthritis*. Oxford: Oxford University Press, 1998:255–61

highly atypical – with OA affecting joints not generally involved in primary OA (e.g. the elbow), with the disease often becoming apparent as early as adolescence and, generally, with clear evidence of underlying dysplastic changes (Table 10). The prevalence of occult genetic abnormalities in cartilage collagen or other matrix macromolecules in individuals with what appears to be typical idiopathic OA remains to be determined. To date, genetic abnormalities have not been identified in patients presenting with a typical clinical picture of idiopathic OA of the hip or knee.

Bone density

An inverse relationship appears to exist between OA and osteoporosis (Figure 8). Bone density in patients with OA is greater than that in age-matched controls, even at sites remote from the OA joint. To some extent, the increase in bone mass in OA may be explained by the association of OA with obesity. It has been suggested that the less dense subchondral bone in osteoporosis absorbs load better than normal bone so that less stress is transferred to the overlying articular cartilage. Indirect evidence to support this general hypothesis includes the finding of a higher than expected prevalence of OA in subjects with osteopetrosis (Figure 9) and in those with greater than average bone mineral density (bone mass).

Estrogen deficiency

Not only is the incidence of OA greater in older women than in older men, but hip and knee OA seem to occur at an accelerated rate in women after about the age of 50, i.e. roughly the time of menopause. Furthermore, some women develop rapidly progressive OA of the hand at this time of life. These relationships suggest that postmenopausal estrogen deficiency may increase the risk of OA. Cross-sectional studies have consistently suggested that women who have used hormonal replacement therapy are at lower risk of developing knee or hip OA than women who have not used estrogen. The reduction in the risk of hip OA among estrogen users has been reported to be as great as 40%. Longitudinal studies have also indicated that current estrogen users are at lower risk for knee OA than non-users, although data from randomized controlled trials are needed before a recommendation can be made that estrogen should be used for the prevention or treatment of OA.

Nutritional deficiencies

Recent data suggest that men and women with moderately low serum levels of 25-hydroxy vitamin D are at greater risk of progression (but not of initiation) of knee OA than those who had a higher vitamin D level. Similar results were obtained in a prospective study of radiographic hip OA, although the effect of vitamin D on symptomatic OA is not known.

Data have suggested that reactive oxygen species may contribute to articular cartilage damage in OA. Because vitamin C is a major dietary antioxidant, it is notable that vitamin C deficiency has been suggested to be a risk factor for OA. Subjects in the lowest third of the population with respect to vitamin C intake, as assessed by a food frequency questionnaire, had 3 times the risk of progression of knee OA, and a greater risk of knee pain, than those with a higher vitamin C intake. As was the case for vitamin D deficiency, lower vitamin C intake did not appear to affect the rate of incidence of knee OA.

Risk factors for progression of osteoarthritis

A variety of evidence suggests that the risk factors associated with the progression of OA are different from those associated with the initiation of joint damage. Several risk factors for OA progression are listed in Table 11. As indicated above, once tissue damage is established, low levels of vitamin C or vitamin D may increase the rate of progression of OA, although prospective studies are needed to confirm this possibility. Weight reduction, if the individual is obese, may have the opposite effect.

Risk factors for pain and disability in osteoarthritis

Most individuals with X-ray evidence of OA do not have joint symptoms. On the other hand, symptoms of OA may be present even in patients with normal joint radiographs. Indeed, in all age groups for which data are available, the prevalence of knee pain exceeds the prevalence of X-ray changes of knee arthritis (Table 12). Risk factors for pain and disability in OA must be differentiated from risk factors for structural changes. Anxiety, depression and muscle weakness may all be more important determinants of disability in patients with knee OA than severity of the pathologic changes. In any given joint, OA may result from a combination of local etiologic factors (e.g. trauma) and a diathesis for generalized OA due to a genetic predisposition, chondrocalcinosis, generalized hypermobility or other factors.

Given comparable degrees of pathologic severity, women with OA are more likely to be disabled than men, those on welfare more likely than those who are working, and divorced subjects more likely than those who are married. The factors that determine why and when a person with X-ray features of OA decides to seek medical attention are poorly understood, but may be related to the individual's framework of social support and coping skills.

Bibliography

Felson DT. Preventing knee and hip osteoarthritis. *Bull Rheum Dis* 1998;47:1–8

Felson DT, Anderson JJ, Naimark A, et al. Obesity and knee osteoarthritis: the Framingham Study. *Ann Intern Med* 1988;109:18–24

Felson DT, Zhang Y, Anthony JM, et al. Weight loss reduces the risk for symptomatic knee osteoarthritis in women. *Ann Intern Med* 1992;116:535–9

Guccione AA, Felson DT, Anderson JJ, et al. The effects of specific medical conditions on the functional limitations of elders in the Framingham Study. *Am J Public Health* 1994;84:351–8

Hadler N. Why does the patient with osteoarthritis hurt? In Brandt KD, Doherty M, Lohmander SL, eds. *Textbook of Osteoarthritis.* Oxford: Oxford University Press, 1998;255–61

Lane NE, Michel B, Bjorkengren A, et al. The risk of osteoarthritis with running and aging: a 5-year longitudinal study. *J Rheumatol* 1993;20:461–8

Loesser RF. The role of aging in the etiopathogenesis and treatment of osteoarthritis. *Rheum Dis Clin North Am* 2000; in press

Roos H, Lindberg H, Gardsell P, et al. The prevalence of gonarthrosis and its relationship to meniscectomy in former soccer players. *Am J Sports Med* 1995;22:219–22

Slemenda C, Brandt KD, Heilman MS, et al. Quadriceps weakness and osteoarthritis of the knee. *Ann Intern Med* 1997;127:97–104

Slemenda C, Heilman DK, Brandt KD, et al. Reduced quadriceps strength relative to body weight: a risk factor for knee osteoarthritis in women? *Arthritis Rheum* 1998;41:1951–9

Summers NM, Haley WE, Reveille JD, Alarcon GS. Radiographic assessment and psychological variables as predictors of pain and functional impairment in osteoarthritis of the knee or hip. *Arthritis Rheum* 1988;31:204–9

CHAPTER THREE
Pathology of osteoarthritis

The pathology of osteoarthritis (OA) reflects both damage to the joint and reaction to that damage. Although the most striking gross changes are usually seen in the load-bearing areas of the articular cartilage (Figures 1 and 2), OA is not a disease of a single tissue, i.e., articular cartilage, but a disease of an organ, the synovial joint, in which all of the tissues – subchondral bone, synovium, capsule, ligaments, periarticular muscle, sensory nerves – as well as the cartilage, are involved (Table 1). OA represents failure of the joint. Just as the heart can fail because of a primary disorder of the endocardium, myocardium, or epicardium – in each case producing a syndrome of congestive heart failure – the joint can fail because of a primary abnormality in the articular cartilage, underlying bone, synovium or periarticular muscle, in each case producing a syndrome which we recognize as OA.

Table 1 Gross pathologic features of osteoarthritis

Softening, fibrillation and, eventually, loss of articular cartilage (although the cartilage may be thicker than normal in the earlier stages of OA)

Eburnation of exposed bone

Bone remodeling

Osteophytes

Subchondral cysts

Synovitis

Thickening of the joint capsule

Meniscus degeneration

Periarticular muscle atrophy

Figure 1 Advanced osteoarthritis of the knee. The joint has been opened anteriorly and the patella has been reflected downward. Note the large ulcerated areas of articular cartilage in the intercondylar region and on the femoral condyle surfaces and patella. Reprinted from the *Clinical Slide Collection on the Rheumatic Diseases*, © 1991. Used by permission of the American College of Rheumatology

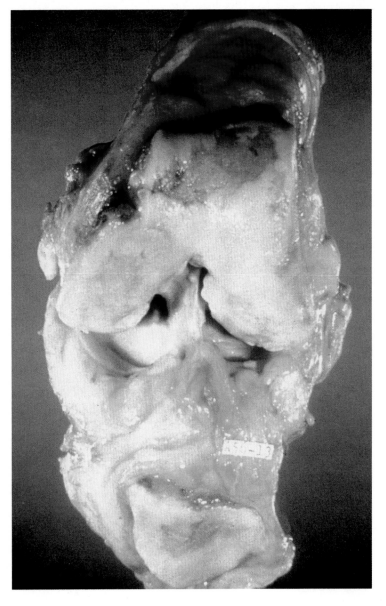

Figure 2 End-stage osteoarthritis. (a) Note the thinning of the articular surface, which has resulted in full-thickness loss of the cartilage over a large portion of the femoral head. A large subchondral cyst is present centrally and osteophytes are apparent at the margins. (b) Femoral head from another patient with end-stage OA, showing loss of cartilage with smooth, eburnated bone, resembling a billiard ball. (c) End-stage OA of the knee. Note the full-thickness loss of articular cartilage, with extensive exposure of subchondral bone and only small islands of cartilage remaining on the joint surface. From Sokoloff L. *The Biology of Degenerative Joint Disease*. Chicago: The University of Chicago Press, 1969:1–162

Figure 3 Normal articular cartilage. Cartilage covers the ends of the bones in every movable joint, where it transmits load from one bone to the other and provides a smooth bearing surface permitting virtually frictionless motion

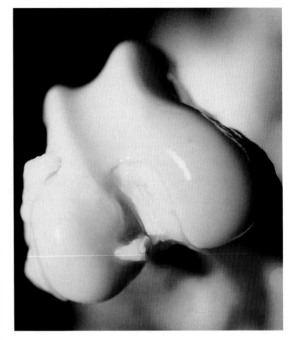

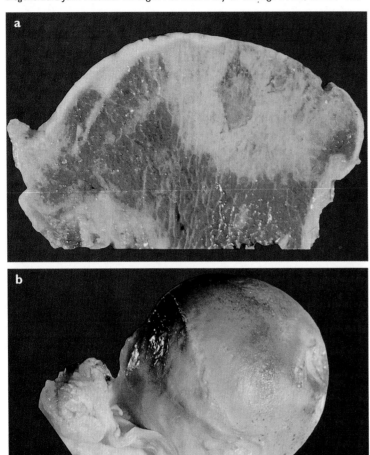

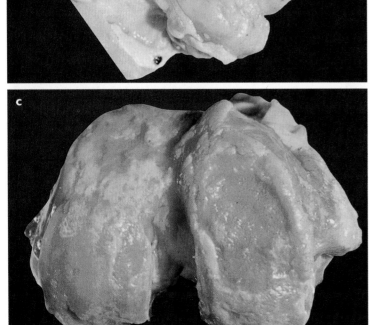

Most descriptions of the pathology of OA emphasize the progressive loss of articular cartilage that occurs in this disease. Indeed, the integrity of the articular cartilage is essential to normal joint function. Normal joint cartilage (Figure 3) subserves two essential functions: first, it provides a smooth bearing surface, so that one bone glides effortlessly over the other with joint movement. (The coefficient of friction of cartilage passing over cartilage in a normal joint is some 15 times lower than that of two ice cubes passed across each other.) Second, articular cartilage transmits load so that, for example, during ambulation, as the femur impinges on the tibia, the bones do not shatter.

In the earlier stages of OA, however, the articular cartilage is not attenuated, but thicker than normal (Figures 4 & 5). An increase in water content, reflecting damage to the collagen network, leads to swelling of the cartilage and is associated with an increase in the net rate of synthesis of proteoglycans, the matrix macromolecules that contribute elasticity to the cartilage and endow it with its ability to resist compression. The increase in proteoglycan synthesis, which represents a repair effort by

Figure 4   Both knees of a dog in which osteoarthritis had been induced by transection of the anterior cruciate ligament 6 months earlier. Note the greater thickness of the articular cartilage in the OA knee (R), in comparison with cartilage from the unoperated contralateral knee of the same animal (L). This increase in cartilage thickness reflects the stage of hypertrophic repair which, in humans, may persist for years before the joint decompensates and full-thickness loss of the cartilage ensues. Reproduced with permission from Adams ME, Brandt KD. Hypertrophic repair of canine articular cartilage in osteoarthritis after anterior cruciate ligament transection. *J Rheumatol* 1991;18:428–35

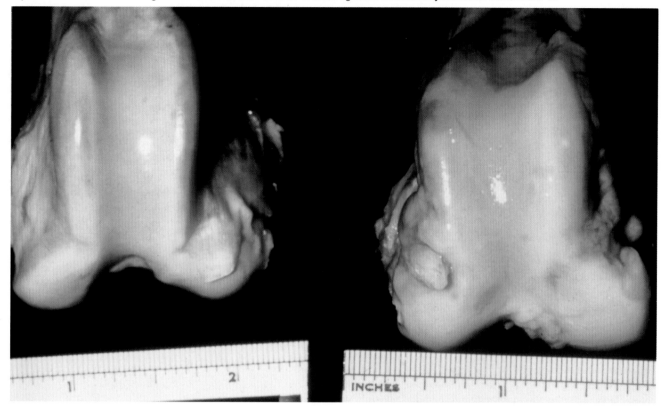

Figure 5   Histologic sections from the central portion of the medial femoral condyles of the knees depicted in Figure 4. The sample from the OA knee (left) is thicker than that from the essentially normal contralateral knee (right)

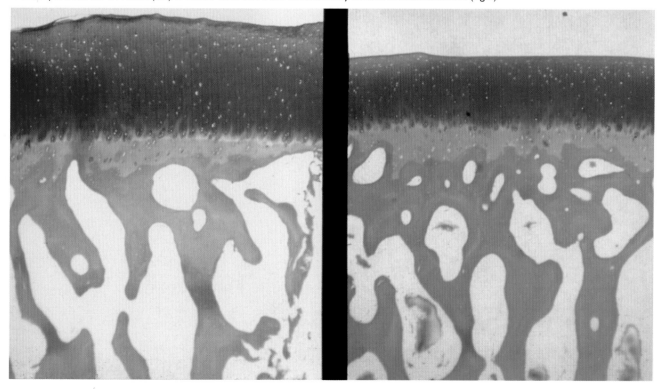

Figure 6 Magnetic resonance image of the right (a) and left (b) knees of a dog 3 years after transection of the left anterior cruciate ligament, resulting in OA. Note the persistence of cartilage thickening on the femoral condyle of the OA knee (arrow), in comparison with cartilage of the unoperated contralateral knee, whose thickness is normal

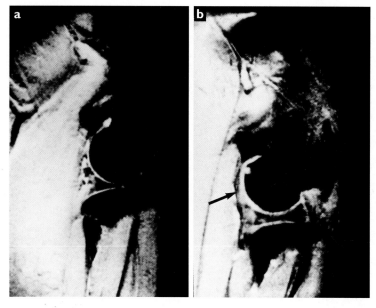

Figure 7 Fibrillation of articular cartilage in osteoarthritis. (a) Note the disruption of surface integrity, with vertical clefts (fibrillation) extending into the depths of the cartilage. Chondrocytes have been lost in some areas. In other areas, cloning of the chondrocytes is apparent. Synthesis of DNA by the chondrocytes is increased in OA. Although cartilage chondrocytes in normal adult articular cartilage do not undergo cell division, chondrocyte cloning may be prominent in OA. Clusters containing as many as 25 chondrocytes or more may be seen as a manifestation of the repair activity in the cartilage. Synthesis not only of DNA, but of RNA, proteoglycans, collagen and noncollagenous proteins is increased in OA. It is, therefore, patently incorrect to call OA a 'degenerative joint disease'. (b) Much earlier stage of fibrillation, before loss of thickness of the articular cartilage. However, even at this early stage, there is some depletion of cartilage matrix proteogylcans, depicted by the decrease in intensity of safranin-O staining around the vertical fissure. Some increase in chondrocyte death is also apparent below the surface, as reflected by the vacant lacunae

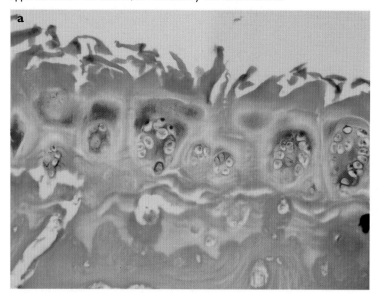

the chondrocytes, may result in an increase in the total proteoglycan concentration of the tissue. Thus, the earlier stages of OA – which, in humans, may last decades (Figure 6) – are characterized by hypertrophic repair of the articular cartilage.

With progression of OA, the joint surface undergoes thinning and the proteoglycan concentration diminishes, leading to softening of the cartilage. Surface integrity is lost and vertical clefts develop (fibrillation) (Figure 7). With motion, the fibrillated cartilage is worn away, exposing underlying bone (Figure 8). Areas of fibrocartilaginous repair may appear (Figure 9) but these are inferior to pristine hyaline articular cartilage in their ability to withstand mechanical stress. The chondrocytes which, in normal adult articular cartilage, do not undergo cell division, replicate, forming clusters (clones) (Figure 7a). Later, however, the remaining cartilage becomes hypocellular.

In the deep zone of normal articular cartilage a zone of increased calcification is separated from the uncalcified hyaline articular cartilage by a histologic landmark, the 'tidemark'. In OA, reduplication of the tidemark is common. As many as 8 or more tidemarks may be counted, each reflecting a discrete event which altered the mechanical stresses on the cartilage (Figure 10). In addition,

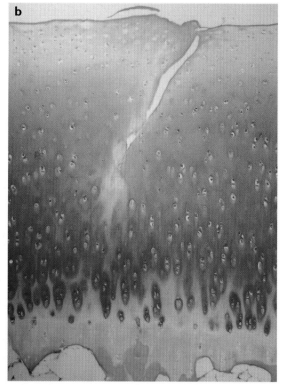

although normal adult articular cartilage is avascular, in OA capillaries from the underlying bone penetrate into the zone of calcified cartilage and beyond, into the hyaline cartilage (Figure 11). This vascularization contributes to the remodeling of the cartilage in OA by providing a route for direct penetration of hormones and paracrine factors (cytokines, growth factors). In addition, the penetration of blood vessels through the bone and calcified cartilage weakens the structure, providing a focus for microfractures extending into the cartilage. Fibrocytes grow into these areas and then undergo cartilage metaplasia and form a fibrocartilaginous matrix.

While the loss of cartilage represents the pathologic hallmark of OA, remodeling and hypertrophy of bone are major features. Appositional bone growth occurs in the subchondral region (Figure 12), leading to the sclerosis that may be seen on X-ray. The abraded bone in the floor of the ulcerated cartilage may take on the gross appearance of polished ivory (eburnation) (Figure 2b). In addition to microfractures of the subchondral trabeculae, bone cysts may be seen (Figures 2a & 13). These cysts, which reflect localized osteonecrosis, form beneath the surface and weaken the osseous support for the overlying cartilage. The cysts may arise by insudation of synovial fluid through microfractures of the surface into subjacent areas of osteoporotic bone, where they may then become surrounded by new bone. Younger cysts contain loose connective tissue which eventually becomes more fibrotic. In some cases communication with the joint surface is obvious; in others no communication is apparent.

The growth of cartilage and bone at the joint margins leads to osteophytes (spurs) (Figure 13), which alter the contours of the joint and may restrict movement. However, in the absence of other bony changes, for example subchondral cysts or sclerosis, osteophytes may be a manifestation of aging, rather than of OA.

Soft tissue changes include a patchy chronic synovitis (Figure 14), with lining cell hyperplasia, lymphocytic infiltration and perivascular lymphoid aggregates. Villus formation may be prominent, suggestive of rheumatoid arthritis. However, in contrast to rheumatoid arthritis, the synovial lining

Figure 8 (a) End-stage osteoarthritis of the knee in a dog 4 years after loss of anterior cruciate ligament integrity. Following an earlier stage of hypertrophic repair, in which the articular cartilage was thicker than normal, repair mechanisms have failed, the joint has decompensated, and full-thickness loss of the articular cartilage is present on the medial femoral condyle and medial tibial plateau. (b) Note the appearance of normal articular cartilage at the corresponding areas of the femur of the contralateral knee

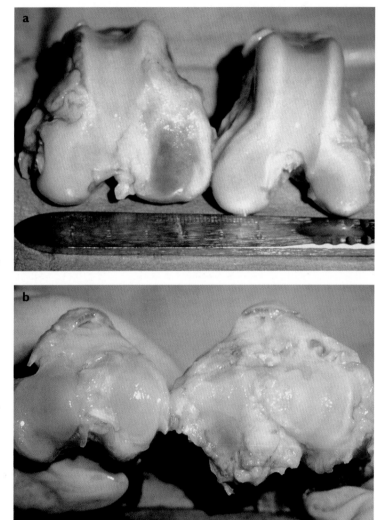

Figure 9 Area of fibrocartilaginous repair on the surface of a femoral head with severe osteoarthritis. The tissue stains very weakly with safranin-O, reflecting a low proteogylcan concentration. There are dense bands of collagen below the articular surface, which is irregular. This tissue does not hold up well under compressive load

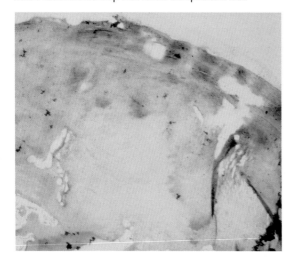

Figure 10 Deeper zone of articular cartilage in osteoarthritis. The hyaline cartilage is at the top of the section and the bony subchondral plate at the bottom. The arrows indicate the multiple tidemarks

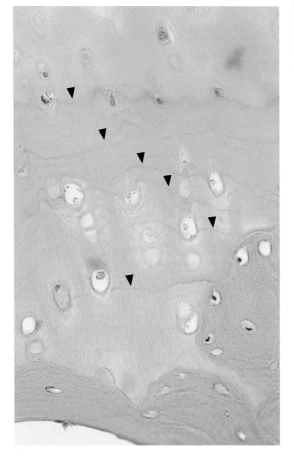

Figure 11 Capillary invasion (arrow) of the zone of calcified cartilage in osteoarthritis. Note the multiple tidemarks, which are seen also in Figure 10

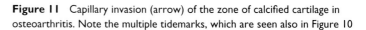
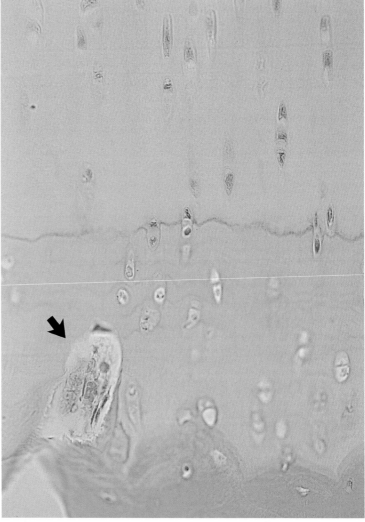

Figure 12 Marked thickening of the subchondral plate in osteoarthritis. Formation and resorption of subchondral bone are both increased in OA

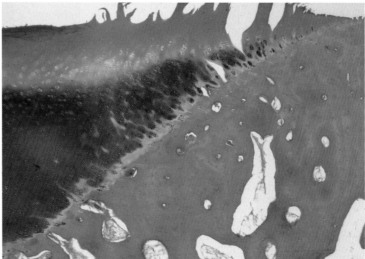

cells do not erode the cartilage at the joint margins or form a pannus infiltrating the cartilage surface. Fragments of articular cartilage and necrotic bone which are lost from the joint surface may become incorporated into the synovial membrane, where they may become surrounded by macrophages, including foreign body giant cells, and an inflammatory cell infiltrate (Figure 15). The presence of numerous fragments of cartilage and bone within the synovium of an OA joint may reflect a rapidly destructive neurogenic arthritis (that is Charcot joint). Thickening of the joint capsule may further restrict movement. In the presence of synovial effusions, loss of compliance of the capsule will lead to expansion of bursal structures that communicate with the joint space. This accounts, for example, for Baker's cysts, which are common in patients with knee OA.

Changes in the ligaments are similar to those in the capsule: dilatation of blood vessels, edema, and increased synthesis of proteoglycans and collagen fibers. Fibrosis may extend to the perineurium and endoneurium, and may provide a structural basis for the chronic joint pain of patients with OA. On the other hand, by stretching the collateral ligaments, chronic effusions may lead to joint laxity. The mechanical instability may result in abnormal stresses on the articular surfaces, causing additional joint damage.

Periarticular muscle wasting is common (Figure 16). It may be due to disuse atrophy, as the patient avoids usage of the painful extremity, or to arthrogenous muscle inhibition, with nerve endings in the arthritic joint transmitting impulses to the central nervous system which reflexly limit the patient's ability to effect a maximal voluntary contraction of the muscle. In any case, because of the importance of periarticular muscle in stabilizing the joint, weakness may be a risk factor for joint damage.

All of the above changes play a role in the clinical signs and symptoms of OA.

Figure 13 Radiograph of femoral head removed surgically because of osteoarthritis. Note the extreme cyst formation in the subchondral bone (C) and extreme osteophytosis (arrowhead). Reproduced with permission from Pritzker KPH. Pathology of osteoarthritis. In Brandt KD, Doherty M, Lohmander LS, eds. *Osteoarthritis*. Oxford, UK: Oxford University Press, 1998:50–61; © Oxford University Press

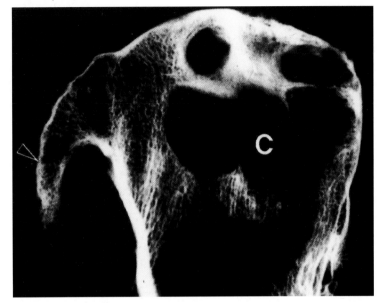

Figure 14 Synovium from the knee of a patient with advanced osteoarthritis. Note the hyperplasia of the lining cell layer and marked focal infiltration of lymphocytes and monocytes. In some cases of advanced OA, the intensity of the synovitis resembles that seen in patients with rheumatoid arthritis

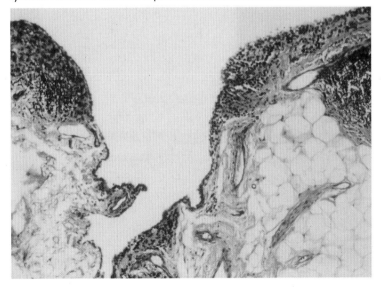

Figure 15 Synovial membrane from a patient with advanced osteoarthritis. Note the shard of articular cartilage, which is a fragment from the fibrillated femoral condyle. The fragment has become incorporated into the fibrotic synovium, where it is producing an inflammatory reaction, characterized by mononuclear cell infiltration

Figure 16 Periarticular muscle atrophy in a patient with osteoarthritis of the knee. Figure kindly provided by Randall L. Braddom, MD

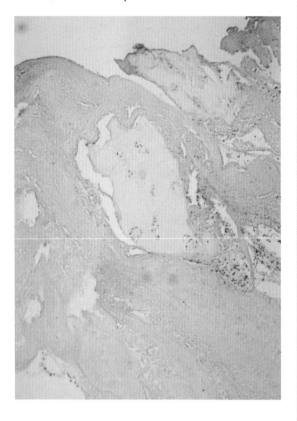

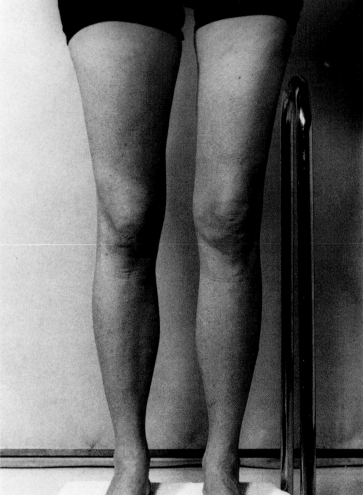

Bibliography

Hurley MV, Newham DJ. The influence of arthrogenous muscle inhibition on quadriceps rehabilitation of patients with early, unilateral osteoarthritis of the knee. *Br J Rheumatol* 1993;32:127–31

Pritzker KPH. Pathology of osteoarthritis. In Brandt KD, Doherty M, Lohmander LS, eds. *Osteoarthritis.* Oxford: Oxford University Press,1998:50–61

Sokoloff L. *The Biology of Degenerative Joint Disease.* Chicago: The University of Chicago Press, 1969:1–162

CHAPTER FOUR

Pathogenesis of osteoarthritis

Although the most obvious changes in the osteoarthritic joint reside in the cartilage, osteoarthritis (OA) should not be viewed simply as a disease of cartilage. It does not represent the failure of a single tissue, but of an organ, the diarthrodial joint. Just as congestive heart failure may be due to primary disease of the myocardium, pericardium or endocardium, the primary abnormality in OA may reside in the articular cartilage, synovium, subchondral bone, ligaments or neuromuscular apparatus. Nonetheless, given the marked changes that occur in the cartilage in OA, it is essential to appreciate the importance of this tissue in normal joint physiology. Normal joint cartilage plays two essential roles: first, it provides a remarkably smooth bearing surface, permitting virtually frictionless movement of one bone over the other within the joint; second, it spreads and transmits load, preventing concentration of stress within the joint (Figure 1).

Essentially, OA develops in either of two settings: when the material properties of the articular cartilage and underlying subchondral bone are normal, but excessive loads on the joint cause the tissues to fail, or when the applied load is reasonable but the material properties of the cartilage tissue (for example bone, ligaments, periarticular muscle) are inferior (Table 1).

Although articular cartilage is highly resistant to wear, under conditions of repeated oscillation repetitive impact loading leads to joint failure. This accounts for the high prevalence of OA in specific joints related to vocational or avocational overload. In general, the earliest progressive degenerative changes in OA occur at sites within the joint that are subject to the greatest compressive loads. It has been suggested that a high proportion of all cases of

'idiopathic' OA of the hip reflect subtle developmental defects, such as acetabular dysplasia or slipped femoral epiphysis, which increase joint congruity and concentrate loads.

Even if the stresses within the joint are normal, conditions that reduce the ability of the articular cartilage or subchondral bone to deform may lead to OA. For example, in ochronosis the

Table 1 Pathogenesis of osteoarthritis

Normal loads + inferior biomaterials, for example cartilage, bone, muscle, ligaments
Excessive loads + normal biomaterials

Figure 1 During load bearing, deformation of the articular cartilage and, especially, of the subchondral bone occurs within a joint (left). This serves to maximize the contact area and thereby reduce the stress (force per unit area). If this deformity does not occur (right) stress will be concentrated, leading to breakdown of the joint. Reproduced with permission from Brandt KD, Radin E. The physiology of articular stress: osteoarthrosis. *Hospital Practice* 1987;22: 103–26 © The McGraw-Hill Companies, Inc. Illustration by Robert Margulies

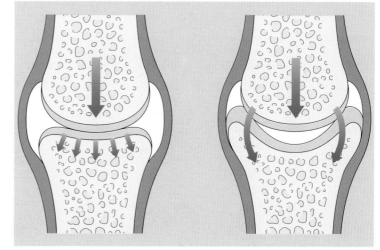

Figure 2 The subchondral cancellous bone is arranged in a series of interconnecting longitudinal struts which transmit load stress down to the diaphyseal shaft. Because this bone is pliable it absorbs energy and protects the overlying articular cartilage from stress during loading of the joint. Reproduced with permission from Brandt KD, Radin E. The physiology of articular stress: osteoarthrosis. *Hospital Practice* 1987;22:103–26 © The McGraw-Hill Companies, Inc. Illustration by Robert Margulies

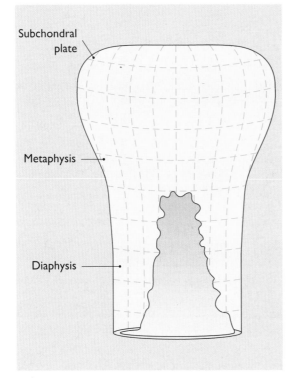

Figure 3 Scanning electron photomicrograph of subchondral bone from a patient with osteoarthritis, showing microfractures. The globular structures (arrows) represent callus formation which has developed with healing of the microfractures. It has been proposed that this results in stiffening of the subchondral bone, leading to degeneration of the overlying articular cartilage

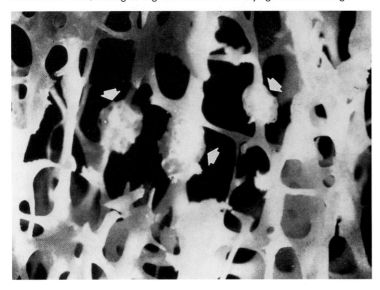

accumulation of homogentisic acid polymers leads to stiffening of the cartilage; in osteopetrosis, stiffening of the subchondral trabeculae, rather than of the cartilage, occurs. In both conditions severe generalized OA is common. Development of OA in subjects with familial chondrodysplasia due to a mutation in the cDNA coding for Type II collagen (Figures 6 and 7 in the chapter on Epidemiology) illustrates the etiologic role which a generalized defect in the articular cartilage matrix may play in this disease.

Mechanisms protecting the joint from stress

The major load on articular cartilage results from the contraction of the muscles that stabilize or move the joint. In normal walking, 3–4 times the weight of the body is transmitted through the knee joint; during a deep knee bend the patellofemoral joint is subjected to a load 9–10 times body weight. Adaptive mechanisms must protect the joint from these physiologic loads. Although articular cartilage is an excellent shock absorber in terms of its bulk properties, at most sites it is only 1–2 mm thick – too thin to serve as the sole shock-absorbing structure in joints. The additional protective mechanisms that are needed are provided by the subchondral bone and periarticular muscles.

Passive protection: the subchondral bone

Normally, in the unloaded state the opposing surfaces of joints are incongruent. Under load, deformation occurs, maximizing the contact area and, hence, minimizing the stress (i.e., force per unit area). Deformation of the cartilage provides the self-pressurized hydrostatic weeping lubrication needed for effortless motion. However, with increasing load, cartilage deformation alone is insufficient; deformation of the underlying bone must also occur and under high loads is more important than deformation of cartilage in reducing stress (Figure 2).

The highly elastic cancellous subchondral bone, although 10 times stiffer than cartilage, is much softer than cortical bone and serves as a major shock absorber. By providing it with a pliable bed that absorbs energy, cancellous bone protects the overlying cartilage (Figure 2). If the load is excessive, however, the subchondral trabeculae will fracture. These microfractures (Figure 3) then heal with callus formation and remodeling. Since the remodeled trabeculae may be stiffer than normal, however, a significant increase in the number of microfractures in subchondral bone may be detrimental to normal joint function. Under such circumstances the bone cannot deform normally with load, the increase in congruity of joint surfaces that occurs with loading is diminished, stresses are concentrated at contact sites on the articular cartilage, and the cartilage fails.

The subchondral bone in OA may have not only a mechanical effect on the cartilage but also metabolic effects: for example, it has recently been shown that conditioned medium from primary cultures of osteoblasts from osteoarthritic joints can significantly affect the release of glycosaminoglycans from normal chondrocytes, in comparison with the spent medium of osteoblast cultures from subjects without arthritis. Furthermore, the activity of the plasminogen activator (urokinase)/plasmin system has been shown to be increased in primary cultures of osteoblasts from the subchondral bone of humans with OA, and levels of insulin-like growth factor-1 (IGF-1) elevated, providing a possible mechanism for the above effect.

Bone mineral density is greater in subjects with OA than in age- and sex-matched controls. Bone formation and bone resorption are both increased in the osteoarthritic joint (Figure 4), resulting in a decrease in the material stiffness of the bone per unit of mass. However, an increase in the number of subchondral trabeculae and a reduction in trabecular separation, and an increase in thickness of the subchondral plate, result in an increase in overall stiffness (i.e. rigidity) of the intra-articular bone in OA (Table 2). Whether changes in the subchondral bone precede or follow those in the overlying cartilage in OA is unclear. However, even if they are not involved in the initiation of cartilage damage, data suggest that bony changes may be of importance in the progression of cartilage breakdown in OA.

Active protection: the muscles

Active shock-absorbing mechanisms involve the use of muscles and joint motion in 'negative work'. While muscle contraction can move a joint, muscles

Table 2 Sequential changes in subchondral thickness and cartilage stiffness in rabbit patella subjected to impact

Time after insult	Cartilage stiffness ratio (impacted/control)	Subchondral plate thickness (impacted/control)
Baseline	0.982 ± 0.17	1.025 ± 0.03
6 days	1.175 ± 0.19	0.906 ± 0.20
1 month	1.005 ± 0.16	1.132 ± 0.27
3 months	0.948 ± 0.18	1.066 ± 0.02
6 months	0.947 ± 0.12	1.416 ± 0.34
12 months	0.718 ± 0.11*	1.561 ± 0.10*

*$p < 0.05$ vs a ratio of 1.0; data are mean ± standard deviation. Reproduced with permission from Newberry WN, Zukosky DK, Haut RC. Subfracture insult to a knee joint causes alterations in the bone and in the functional stiffness of overlying cartilage. *J Orthop Res* 1997;15:450–5

Figure 4 Bone scintigraphy 3 hours after intravenous injection of a dog with ^{99}Tc technetium medronate. (a) Baseline scan; (b) 6 weeks after transection of the left anterior cruciate ligament. The panels on the right-hand side of the figure depict a reference area in the thoracic spine, which is delineated by the rectangles. Note the striking increase in intensity of uptake of the radionuclide in (b) in comparison with (a), reflecting increased bone turnover in the osteoarthritic knee. Reproduced with permission from Brandt KD, Schauwecker DS, Dansereau S, *et al*. Bone scintigraphy in the canine cruciate deficiency model of osteoarthritis. Comparison of the unstable and contralateral knee. *J Rheumatol* 1997;24:140–5

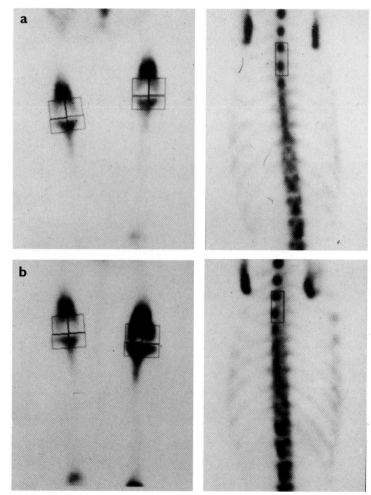

Figure 5 Force trace of load applied to the hind limb of a rabbit with a frequency of 1 Hz. Load amplitude is 1.5 x body weight. In the upper trace, the force was applied rapidly, with a 50 msec interval from onset to peak – too rapid to permit the neuromuscular apparatus to prepare to absorb the load. That impulsive loading sequence led to OA in the ipsilateral knee. In contrast, the same force, applied with the same frequency, but much more gradually (onset to peak interval of 500 msec, lower trace), did not result in any joint damage. From Radin EL. Factors influencing the progression of osteoarthritis. In *Articular Cartilage and Knee Joint Function: Basic Science and Arthroscopy*. New York: Raven Press Ltd, 1990:301–9

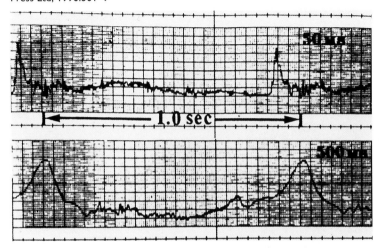

Figure 6 Apparatus for evaluating reflex inhibition of quadriceps contraction. In subjects with knee OA, intraarticular pathology, the presence of a significant synovial effusion, or lack of volition may decrease the strength of a maximum voluntary contraction of the quadriceps, relative to that generated by stimulation of the muscle with surface electrodes. From O'Reilly S, Jones A. Muscle in osteoarthritis. In Brandt KB, Doherty M, Lohmander LS, eds. *Osteoarthritis*. Oxford University Press, 1998:188–96. Photograph kindly provided by Sheila O'Reilly, MD

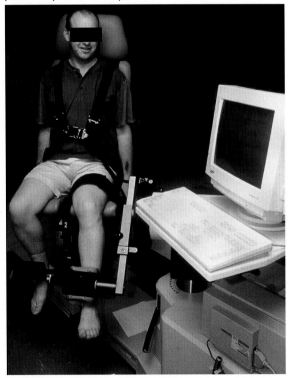

can also act like large rubber bands. When a slightly stretched muscle is subjected to greater stretch as a result of joint motion it can absorb a large amount of energy. Most of the muscle activity generated during ambulation is not used to propel the body forward but to absorb energy to decelerate the body.

If we jump off a ledge or table top we normally land on our toes, come down on our heels, and straighten our flexed knees and hips. During this smooth action, our muscles perform negative work, that is they absorb energy. As we dorsiflex our ankles we stretch our gastrocnemius–soleus complex; as we straighten our knees we stretch our quadriceps; as we straighten our hips we stretch our hamstrings. The amount of energy absorbed by this mechanism is enormous. Indeed, the energy produced by normal walking is great enough to tear all the ligaments of the knee. That this does not occur routinely attests to the importance of active energy absorption (Figure 5). Muscle atrophy (which may occur in association with OA) or an increase in the latent period of the reflex (which may occur with peripheral neuropathy due to aging or other causes) will reduce the effectiveness of this shock-absorbing mechanism.

After a femoral nerve block the load rate in normal subjects, who have no force transient profile during gait, increases more than two-fold (to approximately 150 x body weight/second). This suggests that a force transient can be caused by failure to decelerate the lower extremity prior to heel-strike. In normal individuals, minor incoordination in muscle recruitment, resulting in failure to decelerate the leg, may generate rapidly applied impulsive forces as high as 65x body weight/second at heelstrike. Whether this micro-incoordination of neuromuscular control, which has been called 'microklutziness', is a risk factor for OA remains to be established, but the possibility is intriguing.

While the periarticular muscles serve a primary motor function, the importance of the sensory function of muscle and of the proprioceptive impulses that originate in muscle and are transmitted to the central nervous system has also been emphasized. Data suggest that muscle weakness, due either to atrophy disuse or reflex inhibition of muscle contraction because of intra-articular pathology (Figure 6), may result in joint degeneration (Figure 7).

Figure 7 The role of periarticular muscle in the pathogenesis of osteoarthritis. Reproduced with permission from Hurley MV. The role of muscle weakness in the pathogenesis of osteoarthritis. *Rheum Dis Clin North Am* 1999;25:283–98

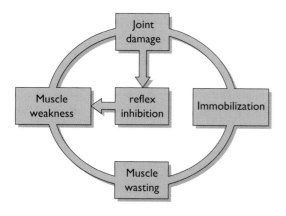

Figure 8 Gait analysis of dogs on a treadmill. The upper two panels show a neurologically intact dog (a) before and (b) after anterior cruciate ligament transection (ACLT). Note the normal flexion of the unstable knee as the paw makes contact with the substrate. This contrasts with the gait pattern in dogs which have undergone L4-S1 dorsal root ganglionectomy (DRG), in which marked extension of the knee occurs at touchdown, (c) is a pre-op study, (d) depicts the dog shown in (c) 9 weeks after DRG/ACLT. Note the extension of the knee at touchdown

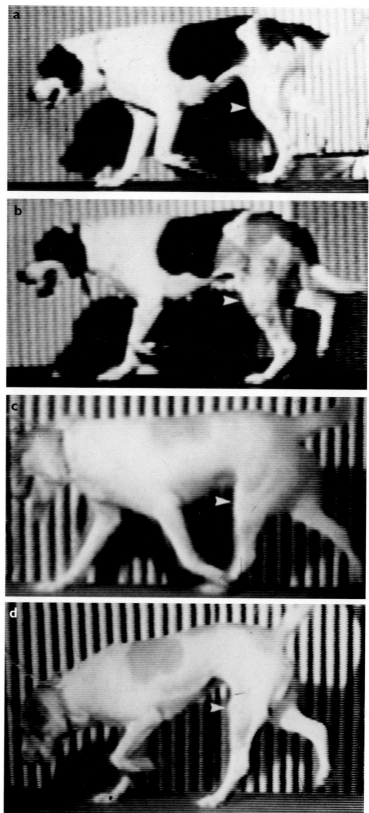

Evidence exists for a proprioceptive defect in patients with knee OA. While it may be argued that impaired proprioception is the result of intra-articular damage, proprioceptive defects have been found bilaterally in patients with unilateral knee OA, raising the interesting possibility that an underlying neurologic defect is important in the etiopathogenesis of primary OA. Furthermore, interruption of sensory input from the ipsilateral limb is associated with a marked alteration of gait and distribution of load in the joint (Figure 8) and rapidly accelerates breakdown of the canine knee after transection of the anterior cruciate ligament (Figure 9).

Recent evidence that quadriceps muscle weakness may be a risk factor for knee OA in humans is discussed in the chapter on epidemiology.

Cartilage loss in osteoarthritis

Cartilage loss is central to OA. The cartilage is slowly degraded, with a progressive decrease in the content of proteoglycans. Because the rates of synthesis of proteoglycans, collagen, hyaluronan and DNA are all increased in OA, catabolic activity of the tissue is extraordinarily high. Although 'wear' may be a factor in the loss of cartilage, it is generally believed that lysosomal proteases (cathepsins) and neutral metalloproteinases (e.g., stromelysin, collagenase, gelatinase) account for much of the loss of cartilage in this disease.

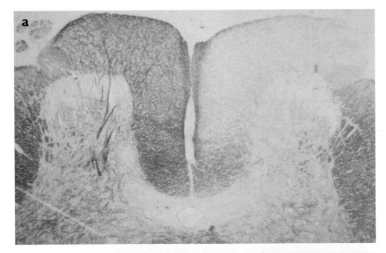

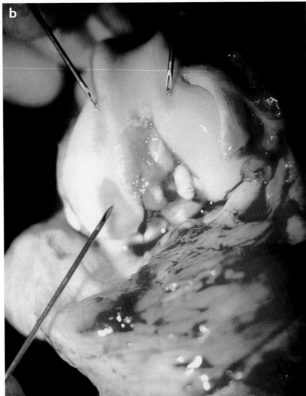

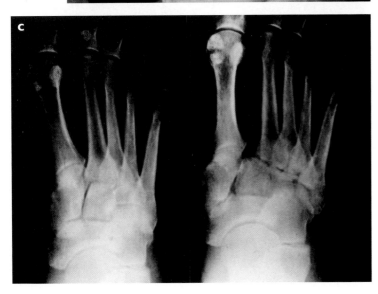

Figure 9 (a) Section of the spinal cord of a dog which had undergone L4-S1 dorsal root ganglionectomy, to markedly reduce sensory input from the ipsilateral hind limb. Note the absence of neurons in the dorsal horn of the cord. If the limb is stable, this procedure does not lead to arthritis. (b) Femoral condyles of a dog which underwent the neurosurgical procedure described in (a) and whose ipsilateral anterior cruciate ligament was transected only 3 weeks before the photograph was taken. The probes point to areas of thinning and ulceration of articular cartilage in the unstable knee. In the neurologically intact dog, lesions of comparable severity are not seen for as long as 3.5–4 years after cruciate ligament transection. (c) X-rays of the foot of a patient with severe diabetic neuroarthropathy. The X-ray on the left was obtained by a podiatrist to whom the patient presented because of a plantar wart. She had no rheumatologic complaints at that time and the X-ray shows no evidence of arthritis. The X-ray on the right was obtained only 1 month later – 3 weeks after the patient had incurred an ankle sprain. A Lisfranc fracture-dislocation is apparent, with patchy sclerosis and demineralization of bone in the midfoot, i.e. classic features of diabetic Charcot arthropathy. Note the analogy to the acceleration of OA in the canine cruciate-deficiency model: in both cases the impairment of sensory input from the extremity and joint instability result in strikingly accelerated joint degeneration

The concentration of collagenase in the cartilage increases with advancing severity of the disease and presumably accounts for the destruction of matrix collagen. Despite an increase in hyaluronan synthesis, a reduction in cartilage hyaluronan content develops, indicating accelerated degradation of the backbone of the proteoglycan aggregate. A specific hyaluronidase has not been isolated from cartilage, but several lysosomal enzymes can cleave hyaluronic acid and chondroitin-6 sulfate.

The slowly progressive loss of cartilage is associated with a loss of aggrecan, resulting in a loss of compressive stiffness and elasticity and an increase in hydraulic permeability. The water content of the cartilage increases and a change occurs in the arrangement and size of the collagen fibers within the matrix. The biochemical data are consistent with a defect in the collagen network of the cartilage, perhaps due to disruption of the 'glue' that binds adjacent collagen fibers together in the matrix. This is perhaps the earliest matrix change to occur in OA and appears to be irreversible. The aggregation defect may be due to an alteration in the hyaluronan-binding region of the proteoglycan

Figure 10 Rapid disintegration of the femoral head in a patient with calcium pyrophosphate dihydrate (CPPD) crystal deposition disease. (a) Essentially normal radiograph taken shortly after the onset of symptoms consistent with OA. (b) Radiograph of the same patient 8 months later, showing marked narrowing of the joint space of the left hip. Note the absence of osteophytosis in this view. (c) Radiograph obtained 3.5 months after (b), now showing complete degeneration of the femoral head. No evidence of infection was present at the time of hip arthroplasty, which was performed shortly after the radiograph in (c) was obtained. CPPD crystals were present in synovial fluid obtained from the wrist of this patient during an acute attack of synovitis which developed at the time the X-ray in (b) was obtained

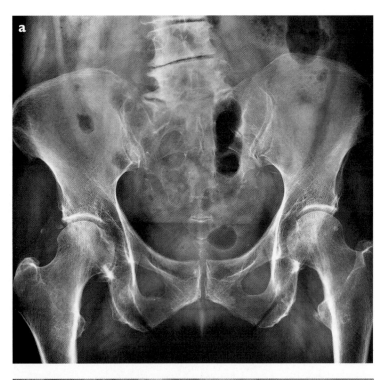

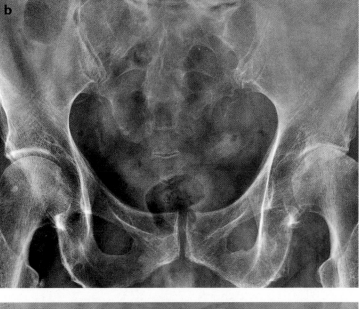

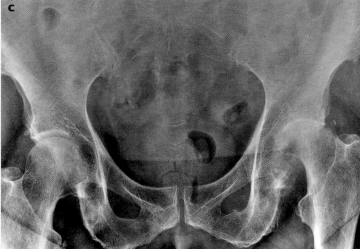

monomer, a quantitative deficiency in hyaluronan or a deficiency in link protein, a noncollagenous protein which stabilizes the interaction between the proteoglycan and hyaluronan. Whatever its basis, it is of considerable importance because the proteoglycans are less constrained within the collagen network than normal. Sites of proteolytic cleavage have been noted in link protein from osteoarthritic cartilage, but are no different from those in link protein from normal adult cartilage.

While the cells in normal adult articular cartilage do not divide, in osteoarthritic cartilage the chondrocytes undergo active cell division. The new cells are very active metabolically, and produce increased quantities of collagen, proteoglycan and hyaluronan. However, the new products do not aggregate well and are not adequately stabilized in the extracellular matrix, so the mechanical properties of the matrix are inferior to those of normal cartilage. Prior to the loss of cartilage thickness and proteoglycan depletion, the marked biosynthetic (repair) activity of the chondrocytes may lead to an increase in proteoglycan concentration, associated with thickening of the cartilage (Figures 4–6, chapter on pathology). This phenomenon of hypertrophic repair is common in the earlier stages of OA in both humans and experimental animals. It is obviously inaccurate to call OA 'degenerative' joint disease.

Many investigators consider that interleukin-1 (IL-1) drives the progression of cartilage breakdown in OA. IL-1 is a cytokine produced by mononuclear cells (including synovial lining cells) and synthesized by chondrocytes, which stimulates the synthesis and secretion of latent collagenase, latent

Figure 11 Milwaukee shoulder syndrome. The rotator cuff has degenerated, resulting in superior dislocation of the head of the humerus, which is no longer in contact with the glenoid fossa of the scapula. Note the bony sclerosis of the upper margin of the humeral head. Other views showed prominent osteophytes on the head of the humerus

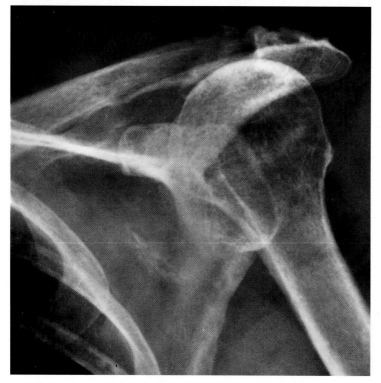

stromelysin, latent gelatinase and tissue plasminogen activator. The activity of the matrix metalloproteinases is controlled by specific inhibitors (tissue inhibitors of matrix metalloproteinases, TIMPs) and by the activation of the latent enzymes. Serine- and cysteine-proteases, such as the plasminogen activator/plasmin system and cathepsin B, respectively, serve as activators. Other enzymes may also serve to activate the matrix metalloproteinases. For example, collagenase-1, collagenase-3 and 92 kDa gelatinase may all be activated by stromelysin-1; 92 kDa gelatinase can also be activated by collagenase-3. Membrane-metalloproteinases localized on the surface of the cell membrane (MT-MMPs) may activate collagenase-3 and 72 kDa gelatinase.

The results of gene therapy experiments offer further indirect evidence of the importance of IL-1 in the pathogenesis of OA. Transfer of the gene for IL-1 receptor antagonist (IL-1 Ra) to the synovial lining of dogs in which OA had been induced by anterior cruciate ligament transection resulted in a reduction in the severity of cartilage degeneration

in the osteoarthritic knee. One month after ligament transection, articular cartilage lesions in joints into which the IL-1 Ra gene had been transferred were less severe than those in osteoarthritic joints into which the LacZ gene had been transferred as a control.

Whether their synthesis and release is stimulated by cytokines such as IL-1 or by other factors (e.g., altered mechanical stresses), the neutral metalloproteinases, cathepsins, and plasmin (which can activate the latent forms of the neutral metalloproteinases) all appear to be involved in failure of the cartilage in OA. Plasminogen, the substrate for plasmin, may be synthesized by the chondrocytes or may enter the cartilage by diffusion from the synovial fluid. Tissue inhibitor of matrix metalloproteinases (TIMP) and plasminogen activator inhibitor-1 (PAI-1), both of which are synthesized by the chondrocytes, limit the degradative activity of the neutral metalloproteinases and plasminogen activator, respectively. A stoichiometric imbalance appears to exist in osteoarthritic cartilage between levels of active enzyme, which may be several-fold higher than those in normal cartilage, and the level of TIMP, which may be only modestly increased.

Growth factors [e.g. IGF-1, TGF-β, basic fibroblast growth factor (FGF)] drive repair processes that, in some cases, may heal the cartilage lesion or at least stabilize the process. These growth factors modulate catabolic as well as anabolic pathways of chondrocyte metabolism. Not only do they increase proteoglycan synthesis but, by down-regulating chondrocyte receptors for IL-1, they decrease proteoglycan degradation. Although the synthesis and expression of IGF-1 are increased in osteoarthritic cartilage, it exhibits decreased responsiveness to IGF-1, which may be explained by an increase in the local production of IGF-binding proteins.

As discussed in the chapter on Synovial Fluid Analysis, crystals of calcium pyrophosphate dihydrate (CPPD) or basic calcium phosphate (BCP, calcium hydroxyapatite) are often present in synovial fluid of patients with OA. CPPD crystals have been associated with attacks of pseudogout and may be recognized radiographically as chondrocalcinosis (Figure 16, chapter on Pitfalls in the Diagnosis of OA). In some cases, CPPD crystal deposition disease may result in rapidly progressive joint destruction, with a pseudo-Charcot arthropathy, as illustrated in Figure 10.

Whether the presence of apatite crystals is a cause or a result of osteoarthritic cartilage damage in OA remains unclear. However, apatite crystals have been shown to induce mitogenesis and prostaglandin synthesis in synovial fibroblasts and chondrocytes *in vitro*, and can induce the synthesis and secretion of matrix metalloproteases capable of causing tissue damage. Their absence from the synovial fluid of patients with other joint diseases associated with cartilage breakdown and synovitis, such as rheumatoid arthritis, suggests that they may have a particular importance in OA and not merely represent an epiphenomenon.

The 'Milwaukee shoulder syndrome' represents a form of destructive OA with some evidence of inflammation in the synovial membrane but minimal synovium fluid leukocytosis. Degeneration of the rotator cuff and severe glenohumeral joint OA are present with deposition of apatite crystals in the synovial membrane. Crystals released from the degenerating tendons presumably trigger the release of collagenase from mononuclear cells in the synovium membrane, leading to breakdown of the articular cartilage, which perpetuates the release of enzymes from the synovium (Figure 11).

Whatever the pathogenetic mechanisms underlying cartilage damages in OA, homeostatic mechanisms may maintain the osteoarthritic joint in a reasonably functional state for years. The repair tissue, however, often does not hold up as well under mechanical stresses as normal hyaline cartilage. Eventually, at least in some cases, the rate of proteoglycan synthesis falls off, the cells are no longer able to maintain the matrix, and 'end-stage' OA develops, with full-thickness loss of cartilage.

Bibliography

Dequeker J. Inverse relationship of interface between osteoporosis and osteoarthritis. *J Rheumatol* 1997;24:795–8

Hill AV. Production and absorption of work by muscle. *Science* 1960;131:897–903

Hurley MV. The role of muscle weakness in the pathogenesis of osteoarthritis. *Rheum Dis Clin North Am* 1999;25:283–98

Jones CM, Watt DGD. Muscular control of landing from unexpected falls in man. *J Physiol* 1971;219:729–37

McCarthy GM. Crystal-related tissue damage. In Smith CJ, Holer VM, eds. *Gout, Hyperuricemia and Other Crystal-Associated Arthropathies.* New York, NY: Marcel Dekker, 1999:39–57

McCarty DJ, Halverson PB, Carresa GF, *et al.* Milwaukee shoulder: association of microspheroids containing hydroxyapatite crystals, active collagenase and neutral protease with rotator cuff defects. *Arthritis Rheum* 1981;24:464–73

Radin EL, Parker HG, Pugh JW, *et al.* Response of joints to impact loading. III. Relationship between trabecular microfractures and cartilage degeneration. *J Biomech* 1973;6:51–7

Radin EL, Paul IL. The response of joints to impact loading. I. In vitro wear. *Arthritis Rheum* 1971;14:356–62

Ryan LM, Cheung HS. The role of crystals in osteoarthritis. *Osteoarthritis* 1999;25:257–67Radin EL, Yang KH, Riegger C, *et al.* Relationship between lower limb dynamics and knee joint pain. *J Orthop Res* 1991;9:398–405

Westacott CI, Webb GR, Warnock MG, *et al.* Alteration of cartilage metabolism by cell from osteoarthritic bone. *Arthritis Rheum* 1997;40:1282–91

SECTION TWO

Diagnosis of osteoarthritis

CHAPTER FIVE

Clinical features of osteoarthritis

Joints affected

The joints most frequently affected by osteoarthritis (OA) are the interphalangeal joints of the hands, the spine, knees, hips and first metatarsophalangeal joint (Figure 1). In most people with symptomatic OA of peripheral joints, more than one joint is affected. Among 500 subjects with symptomatic OA in peripheral joints, only 6% had symptoms confined to a single joint. The most commonly involved joints were knees (41%), hands (30%) and hips (19%).

In patients with hip OA, congenital or developmental abnormality of that joint, for example Legg–Calvé–Perthes disease (avascular necrosis of the secondary center of ossification in the femoral head), slipped femoral capital epiphysis and congenital dysplasia may be present. In contrast, congenital or developmental abnormalities are seldom a basis for knee OA, in which a history of prior trauma, meniscectomy, obesity and certain repetitive vocational activities are dominant risk factors. OA of the spine, which most often affects the lumbar and cervical regions, is not usually associated with a history of trauma. While secondary OA may involve any diarthrodial joint in the body, in the absence of trauma or of a developmental or congenital abnormality, primary OA is uncommon in the elbow, glenohumeral joint, ankle and wrist.

Figure 1 Homunculus showing joints commonly involved in idiopathic (primary) osteoarthritis

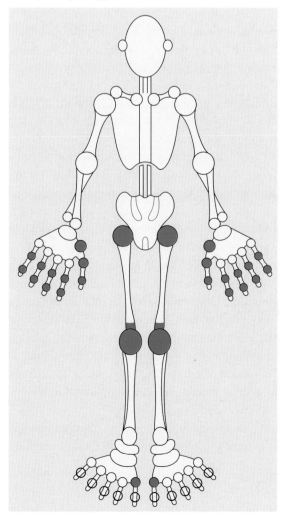

Table 1 Common symptoms and signs of osteoarthritis

Symptoms	Signs	
Joint pain	Crepitus	Limp
Joint stiffness	Restricted movement	Deformity
Crepitus	Tenderness	Muscle atrophy/weakness
Alteration in joint shape	joint line	Increased warmth (±) effusion
Functional impairment	periarticular	Instability
	Bony swelling	
	Soft tissue swelling	

Modified from O'Reilly S, Doherty M. Clinical features of osteoarthritis and standard approaches to the diagnosis. Signs, symptoms, and laboratory tests. In Brandt KB, Doherty M, Lohmander LS, eds. *Osteoarthritis*. Oxford: Oxford University Press, 1998:197-217

Table 2 Clinical features of osteoarthritis

No primary extra-articular manifestations

Usually only one or a few joints are symptomatic

Slow evolution of symptoms and structural damage

Strong association with age – uncommon before middle age

Poor correlation between severity of symptoms, disability and structural change

Symptoms and signs predominantly relate to joint damage rather than to inflammation

Modified from O'Reilly S, Doherty M. Clinical features of osteoarthritis and standard approaches to the diagnosis. Signs, symptoms, and laboratory tests. In Brandt KD, Doherty M, Lohmander LS, eds. *Osteoarthritis*. Oxford: Oxford University Press, 1998:197-217

Table 3 Comparison between radiated axial pain and nerve root entrapment

Characteristic of pain	Radiating pain	Nerve root pain
Maximal over the spine or close to the spine	Yes	No
Related to neck/back movement	Yes	No
Dermatomal distribution	No	Yes
Eased by rubbing	Yes	No
Altered sensation		
hyperesthesia	Yes	No
hypesthesia	No	±
Weakness	No	±
Reduced deep tendon reflexes	No	±

From O'Reilly S, Doherty M. Clinical features of osteoarthritis and standard approaches to the diagnosis. In Brandt KD, Doherty M, Lohmander LS, eds. *Osteoarthritis*. Oxford: Oxford University Press, 1998:197-217

Table 4 Origins of joint pain in patients with osteoarthritis

Tissue	Mechanism of pain
Subchondral bone	Medullary hypertension, microfractures
Osteophytes	Stretching of nerve endings in periosteum
Ligaments	Stretch
Entheses	Inflammation
Joint capsule	Inflammation, distention
Periarticular muscle	Spasm
Synovium	Inflammation

Symptoms: what are the patient's complaints?

In the vast majority of cases, the clinical feature that leads the patient with OA to seek medical attention is joint pain (Table 1). Systemic manifestations (e.g. fever, anemia, weight loss) are not a feature of primary OA (Table 2). Typically, the discomfort has been present for months or years and has been only slowly progressive. The pain is often described as a deep dull ache, localized to the involved joint, which is aggravated by use of that joint – especially, in the case of knee or hip OA, by weight bearing – and relieved by rest. Although the pain is initially intermittent, with progression of the disease it may become constant, increasingly severe and disabling. Nocturnal pain, interfering with sleep, is seen particularly in advanced OA of the hip, in which it is often associated with an effusion of the joint. The presence of night pain in patients with hip OA was found to predict hip joint effusion in over 90% of patients whereas ultrasonography was much less reliable, predicting effusion in only 70–85% of cases.

In patients with OA of the hip, movements requiring internal rotation, in particular, are likely to evoke pain. In those with OA of the knee, extremes of flexion (e.g. squatting) or of extension may be painful. In those with OA of the base of the thumb (Figure 2) or other joints of the hand, pinch movements and tight grasp, as required for opening a jar, may lead to discomfort.

In some patients with OA the pain may be referred. For example, pain due to OA of the hip may be referred to the knee. In those with OA of the cervical spine, it may be localized to the shoulder, arm, forearm or hand; in some cases, pain at these sites may occur in the absence of neck pain. Pain from OA of the cervical or lumbar spine may have a radicular component (i.e., it may be sharp and shooting, and aggravated by the increase in intrathecal pressure generated by coughing, sneezing or straining with a bowel movement). Physical examination may reveal neurologic signs, such as altered sensation, reduced strength, or diminution of a deep tendon reflex, consistent with involvement of a single nerve root (Table 3).

In addition to joint pain, the patient with OA may complain of joint stiffness. Although morning

Figure 2 Bony enlargement and squaring of the base of the thumb caused by bony hypertrophy (osteophytosis) in a patient with OA of the metacarpotrapezial joint

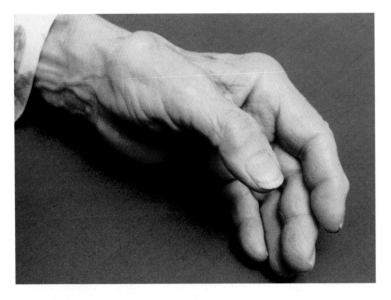

stiffness is a classic feature of rheumatoid arthritis, it is less well recognized as a feature of OA. While the morning stiffness of rheumatoid arthritis may persist for hours after the patient awakens, in OA, morning stiffness usually lasts no more than 20–30 minutes. This 'gelling' sensation in patients with OA may be prominent not only on arising, but after any period of inactivity, such as an automobile ride or an evening in a theater seat. The stiffness induced by inactivity during the day, like morning stiffness, usually subsides rapidly. In those with knee involvement it typically abates after only a few steps. With progression of the disease, however, the stiffness becomes more prolonged.

Patients with OA often complain of crepitus, the sensation of 'cracking' or 'popping' of tissues of the involved joint rubbing against each other with movement. Often crepitus is audible; it is most common in those with OA of the knee.

In other patients with OA, deformity is a complaint. They may note, for example, that one knee has become larger than the other or that the base of the big toe (Figure 3) or a distal interphalangeal joint (Figure 4) has become enlarged. In addition, they may complain of angular deformities, such as bowing of the knees (varus) due to OA of the medial tibiofemoral compartment (Figure 5), or squaring of the base of the thumb due to involvement of the first carpometacarpal joint or metacarpotrapezial joint (Figure 2). At times, the deformity may be striking (Figure 6).

In patients with OA of the hip or knee, development of a limp may be a major source of concern, especially when the disturbance is noticeable to others watching the patient walk. Walking on an uneven surface or on a ramp tends to exaggerate the limp.

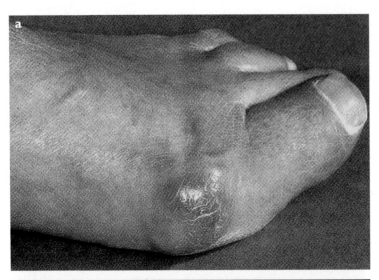

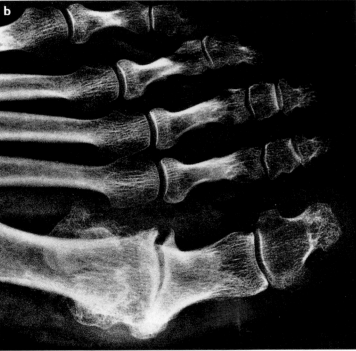

Figure 3 Osteoarthritis of the first metatarsophalangeal joint. This may lead to a hallux valgus deformity with inflammation of the overlying bursa (bunion), as in the patient in Figure 3a. (b) Radiograph showing OA of the first metatarsophalangeal joint. Note the typical radiographic features of OA, i.e. joint space narrowing, osteophytosis and subchondral sclerosis. From Shipley M. *Rheumatic Diseases, Pocket Picture Guides to Clinical Medicine*. Baltimore MD: Williams and Wilkins, 1985

Figure 4 Nodal osteoarthritis involving both the distal and proximal interphalangeal joints. Note the bony enlargement of the distal interphalangeal joints (Heberden's nodes) and several proximal interphalangeal joints (Bouchard's nodes). Gross deformity is obvious in some joints. Reprinted from the Clinical Slide Collection on the Rheumatic Diseases, © 1991, with permission of the American College of Rheumatology

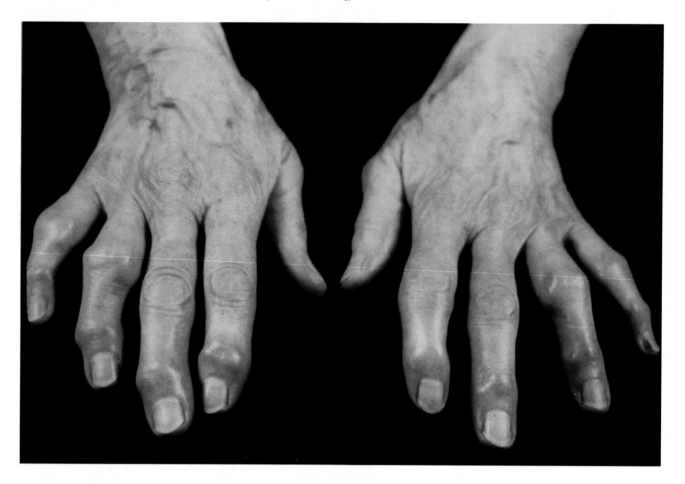

Table 5 Pulse pressure amplitude of the hip, intraosseous pressure of the femoral neck and femoral vein pressure in patients with unilateral osteoarthritis (mmHg)

Site of measurement	Unaffected hip, mmHg Mean ± SD (range)	Arthritic hip, mmHg Mean ± SD (range)	Difference, mmHg, between arthritic and unaffected hip
Intramedullary pulse pressure amplitude	4 ± 2.9 (2–11)	6.8 ± 5.2 (2–18)	2.8**
Femoral neck pressure	18.7 ± 3.6 (13.5–25.3)	48.4 ± 16.3 (27.8–74.8)	29.7***
Femoral vein pressure	11.9 ± 2.5 (6.5–15.6)	11.9 ± 2.5 (6.5–15.6)	
Mean difference between intramedullary neck pressure in unaffected hips and femoral vein pressure = + 6.8 mmHg ($p < 0.001$)			

*$0.01 < p < 0.05$; **$0.001 < p < 0.01$; ***$p < 0.001$. Modified from Arnoldi CC, Linderholm H, Müssbichler H. Venous engorgement and intraosseous hypertension in osteoarthritis of the hip. J Bone Joint Surg Br 1972;54B:409–21

Figure 5 Osteoarthritis of the knee, with bilateral varus deformity

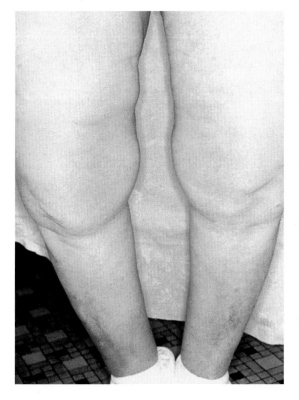

Figure 6 Striking bilateral genu varum deformity in a patient with advanced osteoarthritis in the medial compartment of both knees. From Shipley M. *Rheumatic Diseases, Pocket Picture Guides to Clinical Medicine.* Baltimore MD: Williams and Wilkins, 1985

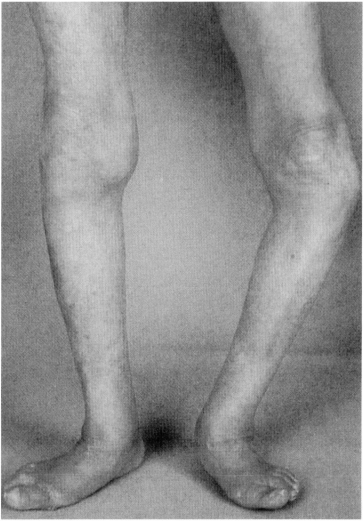

Origins of joint pain in osteoarthritis

Because articular cartilage is aneural, the joint pain in OA must arise from other structures (Table 4). In some cases it may be due to stretching of nerve endings in the periosteum covering osteophytes. In others, it may arise from synovitis or from microfractures in the subchondral bone. In other patients it may reflect bone angina, caused by distortion of the medullary blood flow by the thickened subchondral trabeculae. The latter may increase intraosseous pressure (Table 5) and can cause severe intraosseous stasis (Figure 7). This hemodynamic abnormality is reflected in a prolongation of the emptying time after intraosseous injection of radio-opaque contrast material into the femoral neck (Table 6). The abnormal hemodynamics may be corrected on the operating table by osteotomy (Table 7). Joint instability, leading to stretching of the joint capsule (Figure 8), muscle spasm, enthesopathy and bursitis are additional sources of pain in OA.

Synovium from patients with advanced OA typically exhibits lining cell hyperplasia and marked infiltration with mononuclear cells (see Figure 14, in chapter on Pathology). These changes

Table 6 Emptying time for contrast medium injected intraosseously into the femoral neck during bilateral phlebography of patients with unilateral hip osteoarthritis

Emptying time minutes	Normal hip (n = 13)	Osteoarthritic hip (n = 13)
<3	7	0
<6	6	0
<12	0	2
<20	0	3
>30	0	8

From Arnoldi CC, Linderholm H, Müssbichler H. Venous engorgement and intraosseous hypertension in osteoarthritis of the hip. *J Bone Joint Surg Br* 1972;54B:409–21

Figure 7 Intraosseous phlebography from a patient with lateral osteoarthritis 30 minutes after injection of radio-opaque contrast material. In the arthritic right hip (a) quantities of contrast medium remain in the intraosseous space (arrows). In the image of the normal left hip (b) no contrast material is apparent in either the intraosseous or extraosseous veins. Clearance of the contrast material was completed 30 minutes after the injection. From: Arnoldi CC, Linderholm H, Müssbichler H. Venous engorgement and intraosseous hypertension in osteoarthritis of the hip. *J Bone Joint Surg Br* 1972;54B:409–21

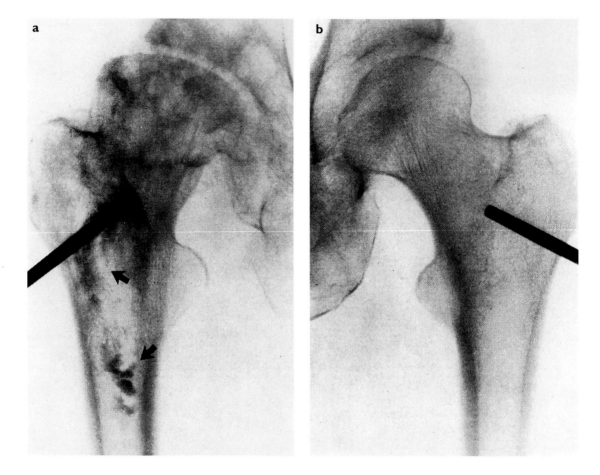

Table 7 Intramedullary pressures, in mmHg, of femoral head and neck in patients with hip osteoarthritis before, and within one minute after, intertrochanteric osteotomy

Site of measurement	n	Before osteotomy Mean ± SE and (range)	After osteotomy Mean ± SE and (range)	Before / after difference Mean ± SE and (range)
Femoral head	7	54.8 ± 8.23 (30.9–88.7)	37.3 ± 7.41 (17.9–61.7)	17.6 ± 2.06* (11.2–27.0)
Femoral neck	7	43.4 ± 6.47 (23.0–66.7)	29.9 ± 5.29 (17.9–61.7)	13.5 ± 2.05* (6.0–23.8)

SE, standard error; *$p < 0.001$. From Arnoldi CC, Lemperg RK, Linderholm H. Immediate effect of osteotomy on the intramedullary pressure of the femoral head and neck in patients with degenerative osteoarthritis. *Acta Orthop Scand* 1971;42:357–65

Figure 8 Semi-thin section of Pacinian corpuscle in human dorsal knee joint capsule (staining after Laczko, Levai, 1975). F, fibrous layer of the joint capsule; I, inner core of the Pacinian corpuscle; C, perineural capsule; M, popliteus muscle. Magnification x 1200. Figure kindly provided by Zdenek Halata, MD, PhD

Figure 9 Histologically normal synovium from a patient with osteoarthritis. This patient had had 3 years of chronic knee pain at the time the synovial biopsy was obtained. Although the knee radiograph showed only minimal changes of OA, full-thickness ulceration of the medial femoral condyle was seen

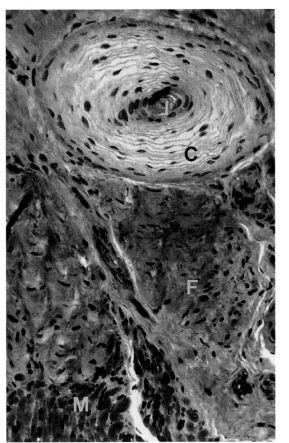

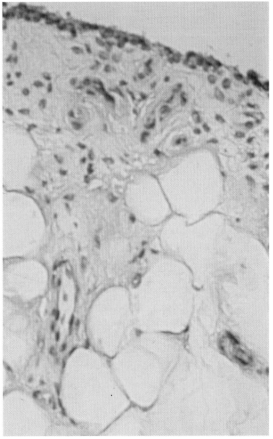

Figure 10 Patients with trochanteric bursitis have tenderness on palpation over the greater trochanter. This figure depicts injection of a depot glucocorticoid preparation performed for treatment of a patient with this condition. The needle enters the skin directly over the greater trochanter. The anterior superior iliac spine and the inguinal ligament have been marked with a skin pencil

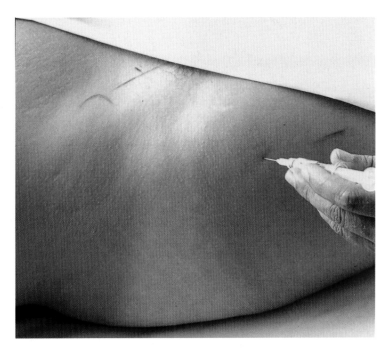

Figure 11 Patient with osteoarthritis of the right glenohumeral joint, causing joint pain and swelling. An effusion is apparent in the right shoulder. Joint aspiration yielded 75 ml of fluid

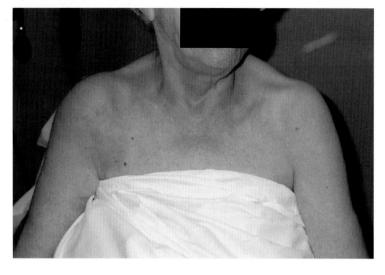

Figure 12 Lateral knee radiograph, showing an effusion in the superpatellar pouch delineated by the opacity between the prefemoral fat (white arrow) and the quadriceps muscle (black arrow)

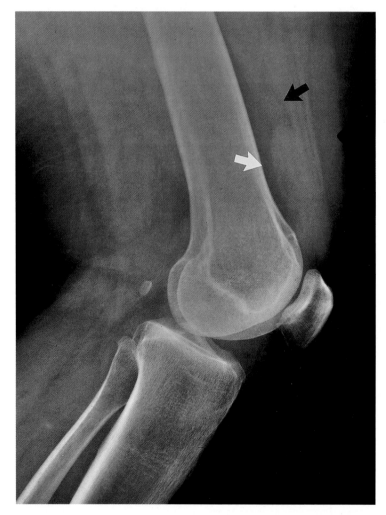

may be qualitatively and quantitatively indistinguishable from those in the synovium of patients with rheumatoid arthritis. Synovitis in OA may be due to phagocytosis of wear particles of cartilage (see Figure 15, in chapter on Pathology) or bone from the abraded joint surface, release from the cartilage of soluble matrix macromolecules (e.g., glycosaminoglycans, proteoglycans) or the presence of crystals of calcium pyrophosphate or calcium hydroxyapatite. In some cases, immune complexes, containing antigens derived from cartilage matrix, may be sequestered in collagenous tissue of the joint, such as the meniscus, leading to chronic low-grade synovitis.

Earlier in the course of OA, however, even in the patient with chronic joint pain, synovial inflammation may be absent (Figure 9), suggesting that the pain is due to one of the other factors mentioned above. Among a series of patients with chronic knee pain who had only minimal radiographic changes of OA, in whom the diagnosis was confirmed arthroscopically, we found that 45% showed no evidence of inflammation in any of multiple samples of synovium, even when full-thickness cartilage ulceration was present. Conversely, the severity of articular cartilage damage and synovial inflammation in patients with knee OA who have no joint pain may be as great as in patients with OA who have knee pain.

The 'joint pain' in patients with OA may arise from periarticular, as well as articular, structures. It is common for the patient with OA to develop soft tissue rheumatism in areas adjacent to the involved joint. For example: anserine bursitis is seen in the patient with knee OA; trochanteric bursitis is seen in the patient with hip OA (Figure 10); and subacromial bursitis and bicipital tendinitis are seen in the patient with OA of the glenohumeral or subacromial joint.

Physical findings

Physical examination of the OA joint may reveal tenderness and bony or soft tissue swelling (Table 1). Tenderness (the sensation and/or sound of joint tissues rubbing against each other with movement of the joint) may be diffuse or localized to marginal osteophytes or to the synovium. Crepitus is characteristic of OA. It may present as the soft crepitus of fibrillated cartilage, as in the patellofemoral joint, or the harder, sharp crepitus of joints in which articular cartilage has been lost so that adjacent bony surfaces rub against each other with movement. This is particularly noticeable in OA of the base of the thumb and knee.

Synovial effusions, when present, are usually not large, although those in the knee or shoulder may occasionally be voluminous (Figures 11 and 12). Palpation may reveal some warmth over the joint. In the advanced stages of OA, gross deformity, palpable bony hypertrophy, subluxation and marked loss of joint motion, often with noticeable contracture, may be striking. Enlargement of the joint may be due to effusion, synovial thickening or osteophytes, which can significantly alter the contour of the joint. Bony swelling due to osteophytes is particularly noticeable in patients with Heberden's or Bouchard's nodes (interphalangeal joint OA of the hands) (Figure 4) and OA of the first metatarsophalangeal (bunion) joint (Figure 3). Periarticular muscle atrophy (Figure 16, pathology chapter) may be due to disuse (as a result of unloading of the painful extremity) and may exaggerate the appearance of joint swelling.

The widely held notion that once symptoms appear OA is inexorably and intractably progressive is incorrect. In many patients the disease stabilizes. In some, especially those with OA of the knee, regression of joint pain – and even of radiographic changes – may occur. For example, Massardo and colleagues described 31 patients with knee OA who underwent clinical and radiographic evaluation on two occasions separated by an 8-year interval. While 20% worsened over the interval and many incurred severe disability, 4 patients (13%) improved and 2 had striking improvement in function. Among 63 subjects in whom paired knee radiographs were obtained at a mean interval of 11 years, only 33%

showed radiographic progression. Notably, pain scores also tended not to worsen. Thus, many subjects with knee OA do not deteriorate either radiographically or symptomatically over lengthy periods of observation. However, it is important to identify the subset of patients who do undergo more rapid progression of their disease and to direct efforts at early intervention toward that high-risk group.

Bibliography

Brandt KD, Flusser D. Osteoarthritis. In Bellamy N, ed. *Prognosis in the Rheumatic Diseases*. Lancaster: Kluwer Academic Publishers, 1991:11–35

Cushnaghan J, Dieppe P. Study of 500 patients with limb joint osteoarthritis. I. Analysis by age, sex, and distribution of symptomatic joint sites. *Ann Rheum Dis* 1991;50:8–13

Lempberg RK, Arnoldi CC. The significance of intraosseous pressure in normal and diseased states with special reference to intraosseous engorgement pain syndrome. *Clin Orthop* 1978;136:143–56

Myers SL, Brandt KD, Ehlich JW, *et al.* Synovial inflammation in patients with early osteoarthritis of the knee. *J Rheumatol* 1990;17:1662–9

Myers SL, Flusser D, Brandt KD, Heck DA. Prevalence of cartilage shards in synovium and their association with synovitis in patients with early and end-stage osteoarthritis. *J Rheumatol* 1992;19:1247–51

O'Reilly S, Doherty M. Clinical features of osteoarthritis and standard approaches to the diagnosis. In Brandt KD, Doherty M, Lohmander LS, eds. *Osteoarthritis*. Oxford: Oxford University Press, 1998:197–217

Schumacher HR, Gordon G, Paul H, *et al.* Osteoarthritis, crystal deposition and inflammation. *Semin Arthritis Rheum* 1981;11:116–19

CHAPTER SIX

Pitfalls in the diagnosis of osteoarthritis

The correct diagnosis of osteoarthritis (OA) is important – misdiagnosis is likely to lead to the omission of appropriate treatment or institution of unnecessary treatment; furthermore, it may be psychologically stressful to the patient. Misinterpretation of the patient's symptoms and signs is a common pitfall in the diagnosis of OA. As indicated above, pain is the predominant symptom of patients with OA and the pain of OA has typical characteristics. Furthermore, pain may arise not only from intra-articular structures but from periarticular muscle spasm or soft tissue rheumatism. The differentiation of articular from periarticular pain is important because periarticular pain can often be managed by local injection of a depot glucocorticoid preparation and physical therapy, without systemic medication. Bálint and Szebenyi have published a clear analysis of the problems underlying the diagnosis of OA, and the factors which confound clinicians in this area.

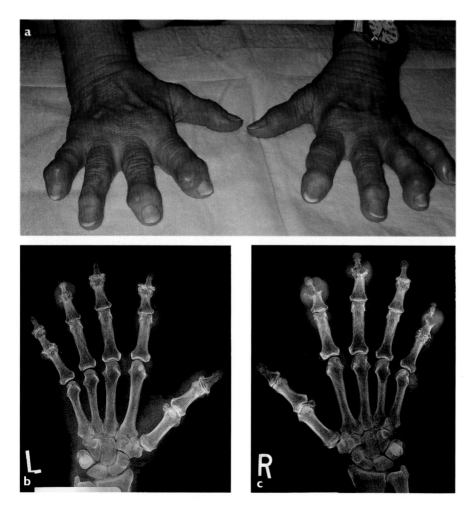

Figure 1 (a) Patient with nodal osteoarthritis in distal and proximal interphalangeal joints who developed superimposed tophaceous gout secondary to chronic use of a diuretic. Note the yellowish discoloration produced by the heavy urate deposition in the subcutaneous tissues around the distal interphalangeal joint. This is most prominent on the right index finger. (b) and (c) Hand radiographs of this subject. Note the prominent radio-dense soft tissue swellings over several distal interphalangeal joints and the left fourth proximal interphalangeal joint, and the associated deposits in bone, with resorption of bone, e.g. in the right second, third and fifth distal interphalangeal joints. Fine needle aspiration of the deposits yielded an abundance of crystals of monosodium urate, readily identified by polarization microscopy.

Figure 2 DeQuervain's tenosynovitis. Note the swelling immediately proximal to the radial styloid (asterisk), reflecting inflammation of the sheath of the extensor pollicis brevis and abductor pollicis longus tendons (a). Figure kindly provided by Alex Mih, MD. Diagram of underlying anatomy (b). Note that the sheath of the above tendons is proximal to the styloid process of the radius and the first carpometacarpal joint. (b) Reproduced with permission from Shipley M. *Pocket Picture Guides to Clinical Medicine. Rheumatic Diseases.* Baltimore MD: Williams & Wilkins, 1985:1–93

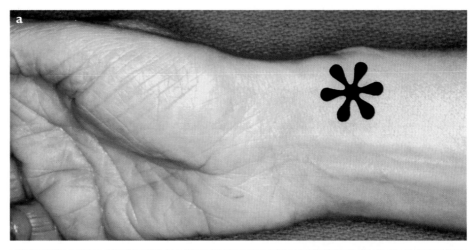

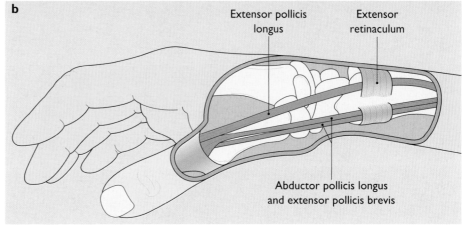

Misinterpretation of pain as a pitfall in the diagnosis of osteoarthritis

Several common circumstances lead to misinterpretation of pain in the patient with OA (Table 1). For example:

1 The origin of pain is not the OA, but some other type of arthritis, trauma, a neurologic disorder or soft tissue rheumatism, occurring independently of OA. Rheumatic diseases are not mutually exclusive: the person with OA has no immunity from superimposed gout (Figure 1) or staphylococcal infection of the OA joint; the person with OA of the base of the thumb may coincidentally develop DeQuervain's tenosynovitis (Figure 2).

2 The pain is caused by OA, but at a remote joint site. For example, pain in the knee is commonly referred from the hip (Figure 3). Radiculopathy due to OA of apophyseal joints in the lumbar spine is a common cause of pain in the hip or

gluteal region. Similar confounding issues exist with spondylosis or prolapsed disk in the cervical spine (Figure 4, Table 2). Localization and characterization of the pain (is it burning? lancinating? is numbness present?) and a careful neurologic examination (Table 3) can help in making an accurate diagnosis.

3 The pain is due to soft tissue rheumatism which has developed secondarily to OA, e.g. anserine bursitis (Figures 5 and 6) or collateral ligament strain (Figure 7) in the patient with knee OA.

Figure 5 shows the relevant anatomy and the sites of the tendinous insertions of the sartorius, gastrocnemius and semitendinosus muscles into the periosteum of the tibia. The overlying anserine bursa commonly becomes inflamed as a result of altered lower extremity mechanics. Hence the condition is prevalent in joggers and among individuals with gait abnormalities due, for example, to back disease, foot problems, or OA of the knee.

Figure 3 Dermatomes around the hip and thigh

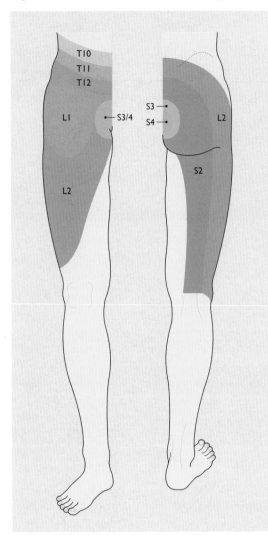

Figure 4 Dermatomes in the upper extremity. Nerve root irritation due to a herniated cervical disk or to osteophytes may produce pain or paresthesias, localizing the lesion. Reproduced with permission from Shipley M. *Pocket Picture Guides to Clinical Medicine. Rheumatic Diseases*. Baltimore MD: Williams & Wilkins, 1985:1–93

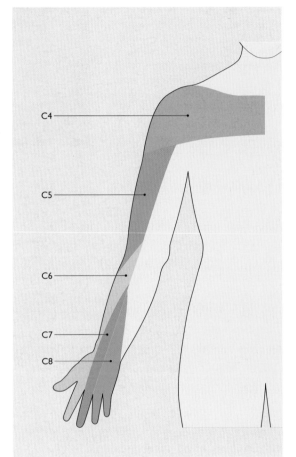

Table 1 Misinterpretation of joint pain in patients with radiographic evidence of osteoarthritis

1 The source of pain is not osteoarthritis, but: • some other type of arthritis • pathological changes in the adjacent bone (tumor, osteomyelitis, metabolic bone disease, etc.) • mechanical injury, pathological fracture • referred pain of neuritis, neuropathy or radiculopathy (e.g. L4 radioculopathy may cause pain in the knee or greater trochanter) • other neurological disorders causing stiffness of joints (Parkinson's disease, upper motor neuron damage, etc.) • soft tissue rheumatism independent of OA (e.g. DeQuervain's tenosynovitis)	2 The source of the pain is osteoarthritis, but not at the joint suspected. For example: • OA of the hip causing pain localized to the knee • OA of the cervical apophyseal joints (C4–5) causing pain in the shoulder • OA of the acromioclavicular joint causing pain in the shoulder • OA of the lumbar apophyseal joints causing pain in the hip, knee or ankle 3 The pain is caused by secondary soft tissue rheumatism. For example: • ligamentous instability (especially the knee) • enthesopathy • bursitis

Modified from Bálint G, Szebenyi B. Diagnosis of osteoarthritis. Guidelines and current pitfalls. *Drugs* 1996;52(Suppl 3):1–13

Figure 5 The anserine bursa is commonly a source of pain in persons with radiographic evidence of knee osteoarthritis. The bursa overlies the insertions of the gracilis, sartorius and semitendinosus muscles into the periosteum of the tibia. In patients with inflammation of the anserine bursa, examination reveals sharply localized tenderness upon palpation over the bursa. Reproduced with permission from Brandt KD. The diagnosis of osteoarthritis: common problems and some contemporary approaches to finding solutions. In Brandt KD, ed. *Diagnostic Studies in Rheumatology*. Summit, NJ: Ciba-Geigy, 1993:1–66

Figure 6 Injection of the bursa with a depot glucocorticoid preparation usually results in prompt relief of knee pain in patients with anserine bursitis

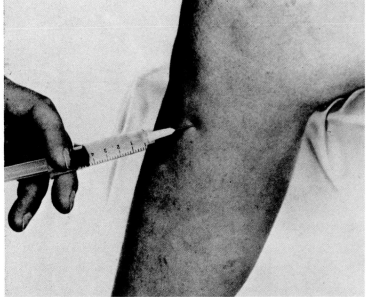

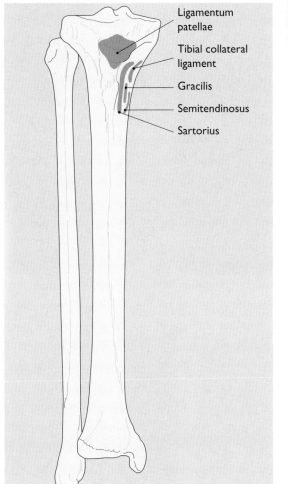

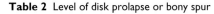

Figure 7 Sites of tenderness in inferior and superior lateral collateral ligament enthesopathy

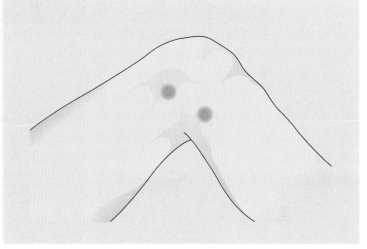

Table 2 Level of disk prolapse or bony spur

Level	Nerve root	Diminution of reflex	Reduction of strength
C4–5	C5	Biceps	Shoulder
C5–6	C6	Biceps Brachial radialis	Biceps Wrist extensors
C6–7	C7	Triceps	Triceps
C7–T1	C8	Triceps	Intrinsics of hand

Reproduced with permission from Shipley M. *Pocket Picture Guides to Clinical Medicine. Rheumatic Diseases*. Baltimore MD: Williams & Wilkins, 1985:1–93

Figure 8 Clubbing of the fingers in a patient with hypertrophic osteoarthropy. This may be associated with polyarthritis. Reprinted from the ARHP Arthritis Teaching Slide Collection © 1991. Used with permission of the American College of Rheumatology

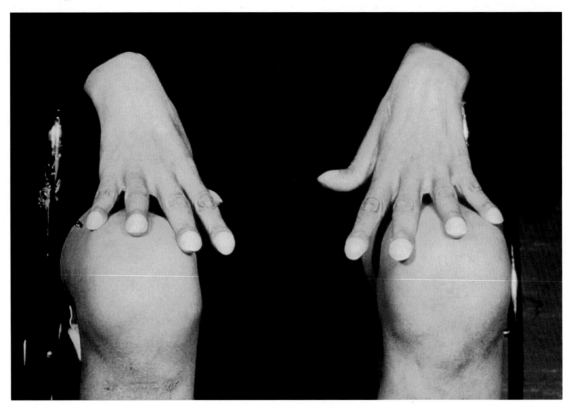

Figure 9 Periosteal elevation in a patient with hypertrophic osteoarthropy due to carcinoma of the breast which has metastasized to the lung. (a) Nodular pulmonary infiltrates, e.g., above the left diaphragm, at the hilum and peripherally over the left, sixth rib. In (b) and (c) note the marked periosteal reaction in the femur

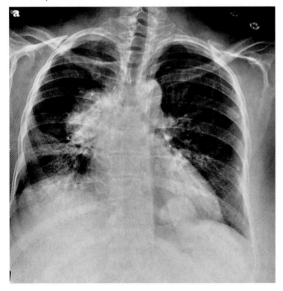

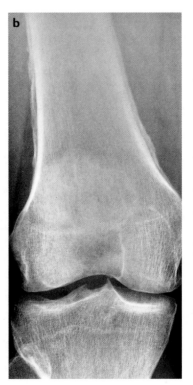

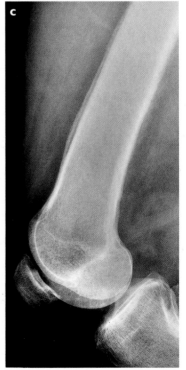

Misinterpretation of deformity as a pitfall in the diagnosis of osteoarthritis

In OA, deformity is due to destruction of joint tissues, such as the articular cartilage and menisci, bony remodeling, osteophyte formation and ligamentous damage. Deformities caused by diseases other than OA, some of which may – like OA – cause joint pain, gelling after periods of immobility, limitation of movement, crepitus and bony swelling, may lead to misdiagnosis. For example hypertrophic osteoarthropathy may be confused with nodal OA of the fingers. However, clubbing of the nails (Figure 8) and radiographic evidence of periostitis (Figure 9) differentiate this condition from OA.

In patients with psoriatic arthritis of the distal interphalangeal joint, nail changes (Figure 10) and skin lesions of psoriasis can establish the diagnosis. The skin lesions may be limited to the scalp line, perianal region, umbilicus or external auditory canal and, hence, require a careful and extensive examination of the integument for their detection.

Flexion contractures of joints – particularly of the fingers, knees and hips – in elderly people may be erroneously attributed to OA when they are, in

Table 3 Level of disk prolapse or bony spur

Level of disc	Nerve root	Reduced reflex	Reduced power	Pain/ paraesthesia
L3–4	L4	Knee	Knee extension (quadriceps)	Anterolateral thigh and medial calf
L4–5	L5	None	Dorsiflexion of great toe	Lateral calf
L5–S1	S1	Ankle	Plantar flexion (gastrocnemius)	Lateral foot and back of calf

Reproduced with permission from Shipley M. *Pocket Picture Guides to Clinical Medicine. Rheumatic Diseases.* Baltimore MD: Williams & Wilkins, 1985:1–93

Figure 10 (a) Psoriatic nail changes with swelling of the distal interphalangeal joint in a patient with psoriatic arthritis. The distal portion of the nail has separated from the bone. Fragmentation of the nail is apparent. (b) Hand of another patient with psoriatic arthritis, showing hyperkeratotic plaques in the skin on the dorsum of the hand, prominent swelling of the distal interphalangeal joint of the index finger, and psoriatic changes in the adjacent nail. Reprinted from the ARHP Arthritis Teaching Slide Collection © 1991. Used with permission of the American College of Rheumatology

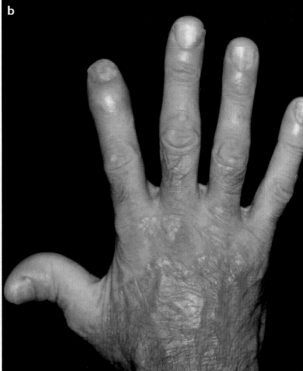

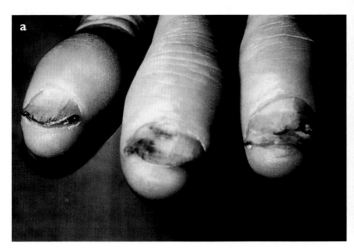

Figure 11 Dupuytren's contracture. Note the thick fibrous band in the palmar fascia, causing flexion contracture of the fourth and fifth digits. Figure kindly provided by Alex Mih, MD

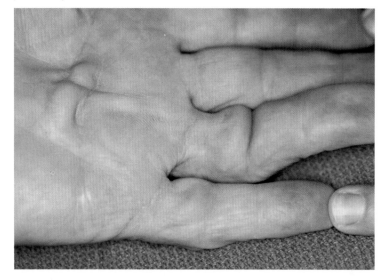

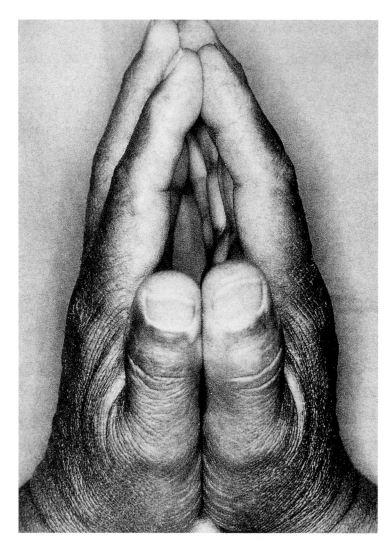

fact, due to Dupuytren's contracture (Figure 11), diabetic cheirarthropathy (Figure 12), trauma or a neurologic condition. Flexion contracture of the knee may be caused by a loose body; flexion contracture of the hip may be due to osteonecrosis (avascular necrosis) of the femoral head (Figure 13).

Neuropathic arthropathy (Charcot joint) (Figure 14) can mimic OA. Extensive periarticular ossification, ligamentous laxity and severe deformity, with marked bony hypertrophy and, often, osteochondral fractures, are characteristic, and differentiate this condition from OA. Although neuropathic joint disease may be relatively painless, it is not uncommon for the neuropathic joint to be severely painful and to exhibit acute signs of inflammation, raising concern about the presence of septic arthritis. Careful neurologic examination (with particular attention paid to improvement of position sense) is important in evaluating a patient suspected of having this disorder. Arthrocentesis, with careful analysis of the synovial fluid, including a Gram stain and culture, may be required to exclude acute bacterial joint infection.

Misinterpretation of the radiograph as a pitfall in the diagnosis of osteoarthritis

Radiographs must be interpreted in the context of the patient's history and physical findings. Misinterpretation of the radiograph is a common pitfall leading to erroneous diagnosis in patients with OA (Table 4). For example:

1 The patient with radiographic evidence of OA may present with a history and physical examination which indicate a second type of arthritis having no distinguishing radiographic characteristics at the time of presentation (e.g. acute gout or pseudogout without radiographic evidence of a tophus or chondrocalcinosis, respectively; or

Figure 12 Prayer sign in a patient with limited joint mobility due to diabetes mellitus. The patient is unable to bring his fingers and palms together because of contractures of the metacarpophalangeal, proximal interphalangeal and distal interphalangeal joints. Typically, the contractures begin with the fifth digit and progress radially. Reproduced with permission from Kapoor A, Sibbitt WL. Contractures in diabetes mellitus: the syndrome of limited joint mobility. *Semin Arthritis Rheum* 1989;18:168–80

Table 4 Conditions leading to misinterpretation of the radiograph, resulting in misdiagnosis of osteoarthritis

> Some other type of arthritis occurring in a joint with previous OA changes
>
> Absence of radiographic changes in the initial stages of OA
>
> Diffuse idiopathic skeletal hyperostosis (DISH)
>
> Joint flexion contracture causing loss of joint space width that is misinterpreted as thinning of the articular cartilage
>
> Neurogenic and metabolic arthropathies

Modified from Bálint G, Szebenyi B. Diagnosis of osteoarthritis. Guidelines and current pitfalls. *Drugs* 1996;52(Suppl 3):1–13

Figure 13 Osteonecrosis (avascular necrosis) of the hip. Note the slight flattening of the femoral head and patchy sclerosis and demineralization. The arrow points to an area of increased bony density, reflecting collapse and condensation of the subchondral bone

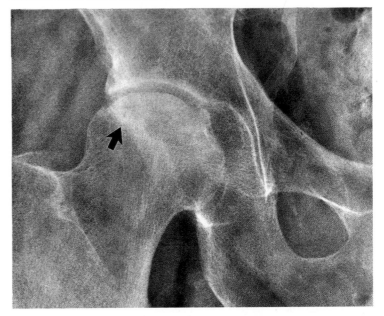

Figure 14 Neuropathic joint (Charcot arthropathy) in a patient with tabes dorsalis. (a) Severe destructive changes in both knees. The joints are unstable and dislocated. Varus, valgus or recurvatum deformity may be present. (b) Lateral knee radiograph of a patient with Charcot arthropathy, showing erosion and irregularity of the joint surfaces, extensive new bone formation and soft tissue calcification and ossification. A massive amount of new bone extends anteriorly and superiorly from the anterior articulating surface of the tibia. Abundant joint detritus is present. Reprinted from the ARHP Arthritis Teaching Slide Collection © 1991. Used with permission of the American College of Rheumatology

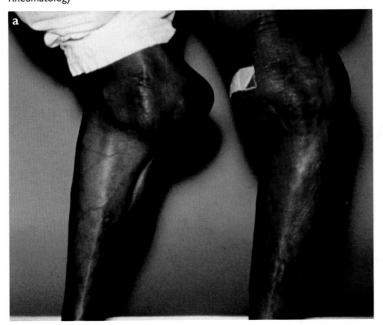

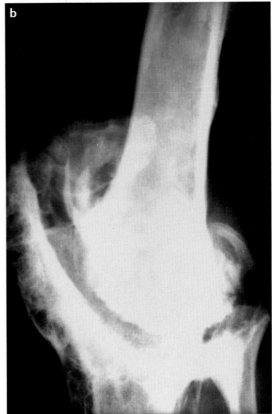

Figure 15 (a) Diffuse idiopathic skeletal hyperostosis (DISH), with prominent ossification of the anterior longitudinal ligament of the spine. (b) Osteophytes at the margins of the vertebral bodies in spondylosis. Note the difference between this and ossification of the ligament in DISH. The histologic specimen (c) clearly shows the anatomic origin of the vertebral spurs

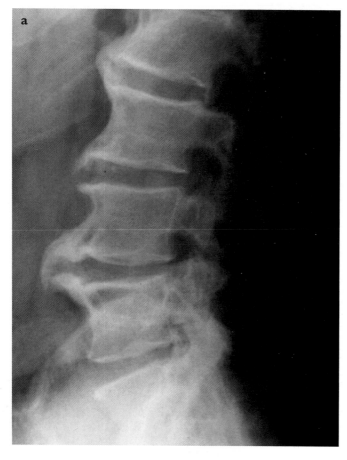

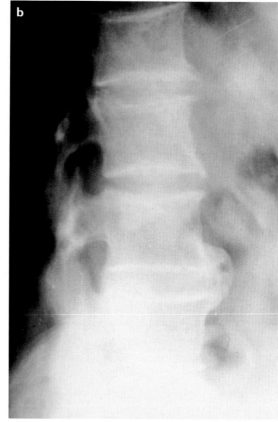

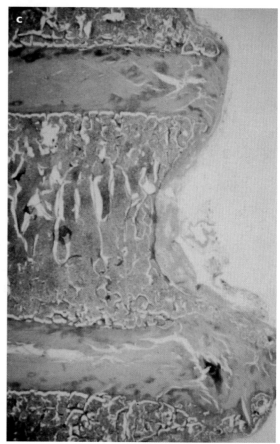

acute bacterial joint infection before juxta-articular osteoporosis and destruction of the cortical margins have developed).

2 Flexion of the knee, due to pain, may result in narrowing of joint space width on the conventional standing anteroposterior radiograph, which is misinterpreted as a loss of articular cartilage when, in fact, the joint is normal and the reduction in inter-bone distance is due only to the position of the joint.

3 The patient may have diffuse idiopathic skeletal hyperostosis (DISH) (Figure 15), with ossification of the anterior spinal ligament, which is misinterpreted as vertebral osteophytosis.

4 The patient may have a systemic metabolic abnormality, e.g. Wilson's disease, hemochromatosis or chondrocalcinosis (Figure 16), producing

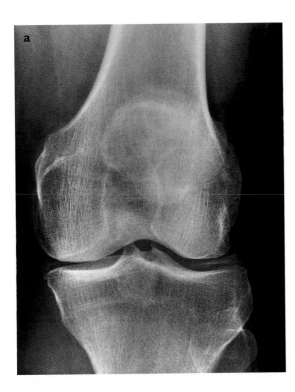

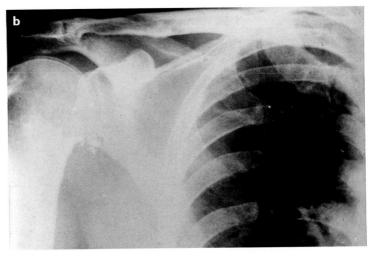

Figure 16 Chrondrocalcinosis. (a) Note deposits of calcium pyrophosphate dihydrate in the menisci and articular cartilage of this patient with OA. (b) Note the layer of calcification in the head of the humerus of this patient with chrondrocalcinosis, who reported acute attacks of shoulder pain and swelling 2–3 times per year and from whom crystals of calcium pyrophosphate dihydrate (CPPD) were identified in synovial fluid during an acute attack of knee pain and swelling due to pseudogout

Figure 17 Rickets. This 30-month-old girl exhibits progressive bowing of the legs and complained of bilateral thigh pain. She has striking genu varum deformities due to nutritional rickets, associated with an average dietary calcium intake of only 160 mg/day. Reproduced with permission from Thacher TD. Images in clinical medicine. Nutritional rickets. *N Engl J Med* 1999;341:76

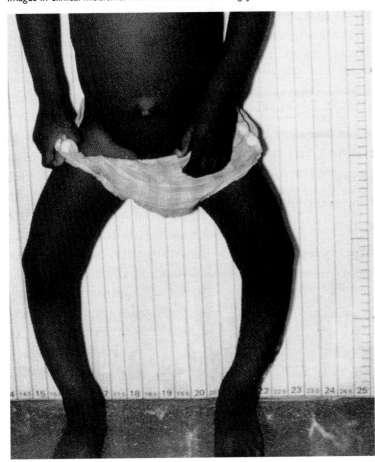

Table 5 Misinterpretation of laboratory test results as a basis for misdiagnosis of osteoarthritis

Increase in erythrocyte sedimentation rate with age

Increase in serum rheumatoid factor titer with age

Increase in serum antinuclear antibody levels with age

Increase in serum C-reactive protein levels with obesity

Figure 18 Femoral nerve stretch test

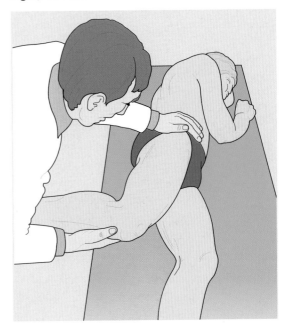

Figure 19 Magnetic resonance image of a patient who presented with pain in the right hip, localized to the gluteal region. Internal rotation of the hip was normal but extension of the hip produced marked discomfort. (a) Shows a coronal T2-weighted image with fat saturation pulse sequence, revealing diffuse edema of the right iliopsoas and iliacus muscles within the pelvis (long arrow) and of the gluteus medius externally (short arrow). (b) Because of persistence of 'hip' pain, MRI was repeated 10 days later. Coronal STIR sequence shown in (b) demonstrates a large multiloculated intra- and extra-pelvic intramuscular abscess in the same areas (long and short arrows, respectively). (c) An image obtained in a plane more posterior to that depicted in (b) depicts the extrapelvic extension of the abscess through the sciatic notch and involvement of the right gluteal region (arrow)

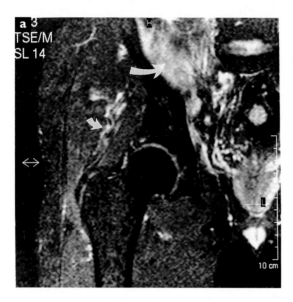

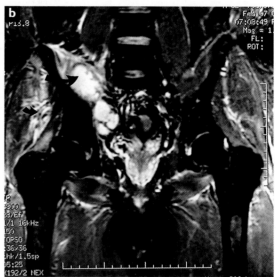

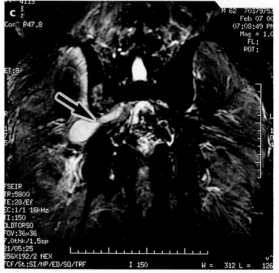

radiographic changes which are misinterpreted as 'garden variety' OA.

Misinterpretation of laboratory results as a pitfall in the diagnosis of osteoarthritis

Among the disorders which must be considered in the differential diagnosis of a patient with OA are systemic inflammatory connective tissue disease and autoimmune diseases, such as rheumatoid arthritis and systemic lupus erythematosus (SLE). Because OA is principally a disease of the elderly, it is important to recognize that the erythrocyte sedimentation rate (ESR) increases with age (Table 5); a sedimentation rate of, e.g. 50 mm per hour, which would be abnormal for a person in her 20s or 30s, is consistent with that expected in an individual in her 70s.

Because many patients with OA (particularly knee OA) are obese, it is notable that a higher body mass index has been found to be associated with a higher serum concentration of the acute phase reactant, C-reactive protein. Furthermore, restricting the analysis to young adults (17–39 years of age) and excluding smokers, subjects with clinically apparent inflammatory disease, cardiovascular disease, diabetes mellitus and estrogen users did not appreciably change the results, which suggests the presence of low-grade systemic inflammation in obese individuals.

It should also be recognized that the titers of serum rheumatoid factor and antinuclear antibodies rise with age. In the elderly, in particular, positive tests, therefore, do not necessarily connote the presence of a systemic connective tissue disorder. In most cases, a careful history and physical examination will differentiate these conditions from OA, obviating the need to obtain measurements of ESR, rheumatoid factor and antinuclear antibody level in elderly subjects with OA.

Avoiding diagnostic pitfalls

Diagnostic pitfalls can be avoided by careful history taking, physical examination of the patient and, occasionally, the use of appropriate imaging methods. These measures are also useful in differentiating the various primary and secondary forms of OA.

Taking a careful history

The key to obtaining a careful patient history involves questioning the patient about:

1 The prevalence of OA in the family, especially in suspected cases of generalized OA.
2 The time of occurrence of initial symptoms and signs. Secondary OA due to trauma, joint laxity, joint dysplasia, osteochondromatosis, osteochondritis dissecans, metabolic disease, etc., may occur at a younger age than idiopathic (primary) OA. The joint deformities of mucopolysaccharidoses, rickets (Figure 17), etc., which can mimic OA, also occur at a young age.
3 The circumstances in which first symptoms and signs appeared. Were they connected to trauma, which may have caused tendinous, ligamentous, meniscal or muscular tears?
4 Previous infection, which might have caused septic arthritis or post-infectious arthritis.
5 Underlying metabolic diseases, such as diabetes mellitus, hypothyroidism, hemochromatosis, Wilson's disease, chondrocalcinosis, which might cause secondary OA.
6 The patterns of pain and stiffness, to determine whether these are characteristic of OA.

Performing a careful physical examination

During the physical examination, one of the most important tasks of the examiner is to elicit the pain which the patient complains of and to determine its source for example, to ascertain whether active and passive movements of the joint cause pain. In many

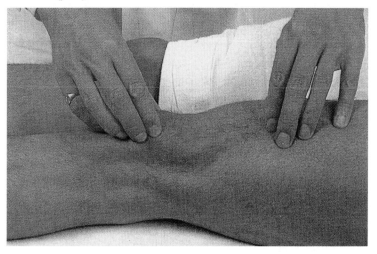

Figure 20 Patella femoral pain is often elicited or aggravated by walking up stairs or rising from a chair. It can be evoked by applying direct pressure over the patella with the examiner's fingers while the patient actively contracts the quadriceps muscle. Reproduced with permission from Shipley M. *Pocket Picture Guides to Clinical Medicine. Rheumatic Diseases*. Baltimore MD: Williams & Wilkins, 1985:1–93 (p. 13)

cases careful examination of the patient will permit the physician to avoid diagnostic pitfalls. For example, when it is referred from the L4 nerve root or femoral nerve, knee pain can be elicited by movements of the hip or spine (e.g. by femoral nerve stretch) (Figure 18). Patients with an iliopsoas abscess may present with 'hip' pain or pain in the gluteal region, as illustrated in Figure 19. Similarly, shoulder pain may originate from the cervical spine and can be provoked by movements of the neck. Pain felt at the greater trochanter may arise from the lumbar spine. Pain in the fingers or toes may be due to an entrapment neuropathy (carpal or tarsal tunnel syndrome) or nerve root irritation.

Pain in the patellofemoral joint can be elicited by pressing the patella against the femoral joint surface (Figure 20). Examination of the knee should include maneuvers to evoke ligamentous, meniscal, or tendoperiosteal pain, and pain arising from bursae. Tender points should be identified. In addition to, or instead of, the characteristic tenderness of joint structures, tenderness of the soft tissues may be present, e.g. in patients with anserine or trochanteric bursitis.

Another important part of the physical examination is the evaluation of swelling and deformity. Bony swelling of the joint is characteristic of OA, especially around the distal interphalangeal joints

Figure 21 A mallet deformity of a finger results from rupture of the terminal extensor tendon or avulsion of its insertion into the base of the distal phalanxes. Active extension of the distal interphalangeal joint is lost and the pull of the normal flexor tendons causes the joint to droop, resulting in the typical deformity. From Labosky DA. Injuries of the Hand. In Radin EL, ed. *Orthopaedics for the Medical Student.* Philadelphia, PA: J.B. Lippincott Co.,1987:35–55 (p. 45)

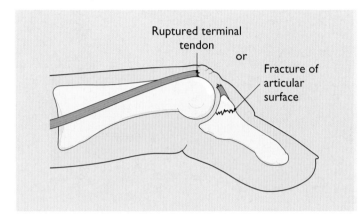

Figure 22 Popliteal cyst. Note the prominent swelling of the left calf. Reprinted from the ARHP Arthritis Teaching Slide Collection, © 1991. Used with permission of the American College of Rheumatology

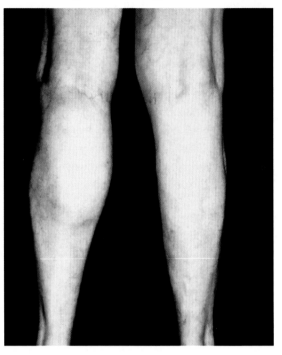

(Heberden's nodes) and proximal interphalangeal joints (Bouchard's nodes) (see Figure 4, chapter on Clinical Features), and the medial and lateral tibiofemoral compartments of the knee joint. The nodes are often palpable before they can be detected on X-ray, because they develop as radio-lucent cartilaginous outgrowths (chondrophytes) which only later undergo ossification, when they may be recognized as radio-opaque osteophytes.

Soft tissue swelling may also be a feature of OA. It may occur in addition to, or in the absence of, bony swelling. Soft tissue swelling and palpable joint effusion are often present in the proximal interphalangeal (PIP) and distal interphalangeal (DIP) joints and in the knee.

Palpation of crepitus may be informative. Fine crepitation felt throughout the entire range of movement is usually of capsular origin. It may occur in normal individuals and has no diagnostic significance. In contrast, coarse cracking felt with movement of the joint may be due to articular cartilage damage, in which case it is caused by the movement of uneven surfaces over each other. One or two cracks felt over the knee during movement of the joint can be a sign of a loose body or torn meniscus. Around the hip, snapping loud crepitus is usually caused by slippage of the iliotibial ligament over the greater trochanter.

Examination of joint function is an important part of the physical examination and may have diagnostic value. For example, in OA of the hip, initially, internal rotation and abduction are restricted, followed by restriction of adduction, hyperextension and external rotation. Restriction of extension without limitation of internal rotation raises the suspicion of other disorders, such as a psoas abscess or iliopectineal bursitis. Similarly, extension contracture of the knee (loss of flexion) is characteristic of spastic paresis, locking of the joint due to a loose body, or contracture resulting from immobilization, but is not usually caused by OA. A flexed position of the DIP joint suggests OA or psoriatic arthritis. If free passive movement of the DIP joint exists, the flexed position is probably due to rupture of the extensor tendon (Figure 21).

It is important to test for abnormal passive movement of the joint due to joint laxity. These abnormalities are common, especially in the knee and finger joints of patients with OA, and are caused by laxity of the capsule and ligaments. This hypermobility may cause a greater problem for the patient than restriction of movement.

Figure 23 Ultrasonogram of the popliteal region of a patient with a Baker's cyst. Lateral view with the patient in a prone position. The skin of the popliteal region is at the top of the figure. The large black area below the surface, delineated by asterisks, is a popliteal cyst. F, femoral condyle; J, joint line; T, tibial plateau. From Brandt KD. The diagnosis of osteoarthritis: common problems and some contemporary approaches to finding solutions. In Brandt KD, ed. *Diagnostic Studies in Rheumatology*. Summit, NJ: Ciba-Geigy, 1993:1–66

Figure 24 Arthrogram of a patient with a large popliteal cyst. Contrast material has been injected into the knee. Note filling of the suprapatellar bursa (top of figure) and extension of the contrast medium distally into a distended cyst. Extension and/or leakage distally into the calf is apparent

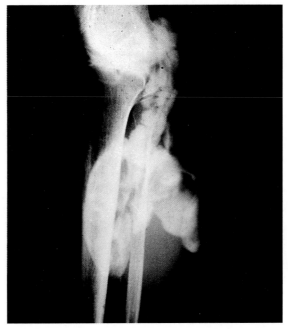

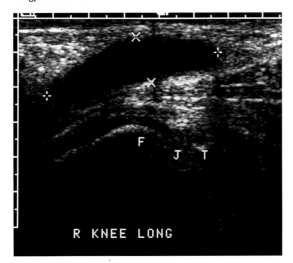

An important diagnostic pitfall in patients with OA of the knee is pseudothrombophlebitis, a syndrome caused by leakage of a popliteal (Baker's) cyst (Figure 22). The diagnosis may be made either by ultrasonography (Figure 23), or by arthrography, after injection of contrast material into the involved knee (Figure 24). The sensitivity of each procedure is approximately 95%. In patients with knee arthritis and a popliteal cyst, a narrow connection between the cyst and the joint can be demonstrated. A Bunsen-valve mechanism permits passage of synovial fluid from the knee into the cyst, but flow does not occur in the opposite direction. Pressure in the cyst may exceed that in the knee and be great enough to lead to rupture of the cyst wall. In most cases, popliteal cysts are painless. However, when they leak or rupture acutely, spilling synovial fluid into the soft tissues of the leg, they produce a clinical syndrome which may be indistinguishable from that produced by deep vein thrombosis in the calf. The patient may not readily distinguish the pain due to pseudothrombophlebitis from that due to the knee OA. Pseudothrombophlebitis should be suspected in any patient presenting with signs and symptoms of thrombophlebitis in the lower extremity, especially if a history of knee arthritis or clinical evidence of knee effusion is present. In some cases, rupture of a synovial cyst may be the initial indication of the underlying knee arthritis.

It is essential to differentiate pseudothrombophlebitis from *bona fide* thrombophlebitis. Anticoagulation, which is indicated in the latter case, is contraindicated in pseudothrombophlebitis because it may lead to bleeding into the leg, requiring emergency fasciotomy for treatment of an iatrogenic compartment syndrome.

Bibliography

Bálint G, Szebenyi B. Diagnosis of osteoarthritis. Guidelines and current pitfalls. *Drugs* 1996;52 (Suppl 3):1–13

Eyanson S, MacFarlane JD, Brandt KD. Popliteal cyst mimicking thrombophlebitis as the first indication of knee disease. *Clin Orthop* 1979;144:215–19

CHAPTER SEVEN

Synovial fluid analysis

Figure 1 Arthrocentesis of the knee. Aspiration of the left knee is being performed with a lateral approach. The point of entry is 1 cm proximal and 1 cm caudal to the superolateral border of the patella. The lateral approach is generally preferable since the needle passes through a fibrous retinaculum whereas the medial approach requires passage of the needle through the vastus medialis obliquus muscle, risking development of a hematoma and increased discomfort after the procedure

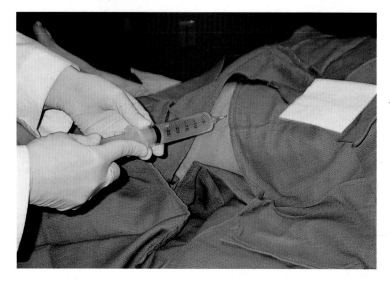

Most patients with osteoarthritis (OA) do not have a clinically apparent joint effusion or have only a small amount of intra-articular fluid detectable by physical examination. Aspiration of this fluid and synovial fluid analysis, however, can be very useful diagnostically (Figure 1). As much may be learned from careful analysis of a few drops of joint fluid as from the study of 50 cc.

The characteristics of the synovial effusion from an OA joint are consistent with the presence of only a low degree of synovial inflammation. Typically, the fluid is clear. It is possible to read newsprint through a test tube containing fluid from an OA joint (Figure 2). The total white cell count is uniformly less than 2000 cells/mm^3 and often less than 500 cells/mm^3 (Table 1). Only about 15% of the leukocytes are polymorphonuclear leukocytes. A good mucin test is characteristic of OA. The synovial fluid glucose concentration approximates that of the simultaneous blood glucose concentration.

Table 1 Characteristics of synovial fluid in osteoarthritis and other common rheumatic diseases*

Diagnosis	Appearance	Viscosity	White cell count/mm^3	% PMNs	Mucin test	Crystals	Difference between concentration of glucose in blood and synovial fluid, mg/dl
Normal	Clear yellow	Normal	<200	7	Good	–	0
Osteoarthritis	Clear or turbid	Decreased	600	13	Good	†	5
Traumatic arthritis	Clear or bloody	Decreased	1500	20	Good	–	5
Gout	Turbid	Decreased	21 500	70	Poor	Monosodium urate	11
Pseudogout	Slightly turbid	Slightly decreased	14 200	68	Fair	Calcium pyrophosphate dihydrate (CPPD)	–
Rheumatoid arthritis	Turbid	Decreased	1900	66	Fair–poor	Cholesterol (rare)	30
Acute bacterial joint infection	Very turbid	Decreased	80 000	90	Poor	–	91

*Modified from reference 1. Data on samples from normal subjects are from reference 2 and other data are compiled from references 3 and 4. †As many as 70% of fluids from patients with OA contain crystals of CPPD and/or calcium hydroxyapatite, or both. PMNs, polymorphonuclear leukocytes

The real value of synovial fluid analysis in the patient with a joint effusion and radiographic evidence of OA lies in its ability to reveal additional, coexisting joint pathology. Thus, a synovial fluid leukocyte count in excess of 2000 cells/mm^3 – even if the joint exhibits classical radiographic findings of OA – indicates the presence of some inflammatory joint disease in addition to OA.

Polarization microscopy of fluid obtained from an OA joint may reveal crystals of monosodium urate (Figure 3) or calcium pyrophosphate dihydrate (Figure 4), leading to a diagnosis of gout or pseudogout, respectively. In other cases very weakly birefringent crystals of calcium hydroxyapatite may be present (Figure 5). These can easily be visualized with an Alizarin red stain of the fluid. Apatite crystals may be an incidental finding, but occasionally are seen in synovial fluid from patients with rapidly progressive OA who undergo very rapid loss of cartilage, as seen by accelerated joint space narrowing in the radiograph. Occasionally, cholesterol crystals may be seen. These are most commonly found in chronic effusions and are asymptomatic (Figure 6). Bacteria may be seen in the Gram stain (Figure 7) or culture of fluid from the OA joint, providing definite evidence of acute bacterial joint infection. At times, examination of a Wright–Giemsa stain of the synovial fluid may reveal the presence of LE cells in patients who have idiopathic or drug-induced systemic lupus erythematosus (Figure 8). Finally, it is important to exclude artifacts, such as talc crystals from the gloves of the physician performing the aspiration (Figure 9).

In addition to the value of synovial fluid analysis in establishing a diagnosis of OA, the procedure may be very helpful in the patient already known to have OA in whom the development of a new effusion or an increase in joint pain require explanation. In such instances, whenever the cause of the joint effusion is not certain, arthrocentesis and synovial fluid analysis should be performed.

Figure 3 (a) Intracellular and extracellular needle- and rod-shaped crystals of monosodium urate in synovial fluid from a patient with gout, viewed under ordinary light x400. (b) The same crystals viewed under compensated polarized light, showing the characteristic strongly negative birefringence of the urate crystal. Wet preparation, compensated polarized light x400. Reproduced with permission from Schumacher HR, Reginato AJ. *Atlas of Synovial Fluid Analysis and Crystal Identification.* Philadelphia: Lea & Febiger, 1991

Figure 2 Gross appearance of synovial fluid from a patient with osteoarthritis, compared to that of synovial fluid from a patient with rheumatoid arthritis and with distilled water. From left to right: distilled water; the sample from the patient with OA; and the sample from the patient with rheumatoid arthritis. Note that the synovial fluid from the patient with OA, which has a low total leukocyte count, is clear; it is possible to read newsprint through the test tube. In contrast, synovial fluid from the patient with rheumatoid arthritis, in which the leukocyte count was 17 500 cells/mm^3, is turbid

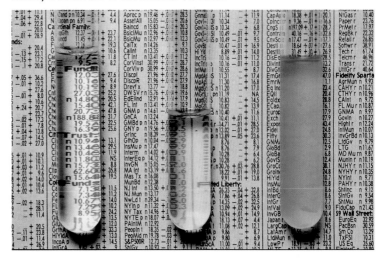

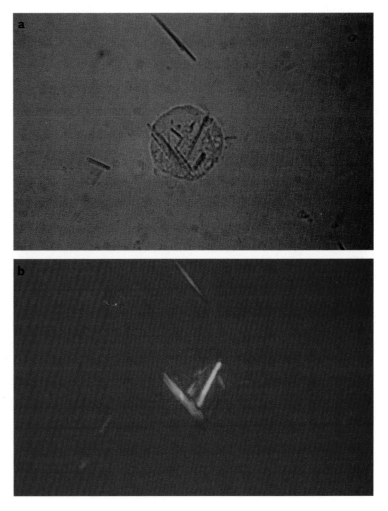

Figure 4 (a) Rod-shaped crystals of calcium pyrophosphate dihydrate (CPPD) in synovial fluid from a patient with pseudogout, seen under ordinary light microscopy with a low condenser, x400. The round bodies in this sample of synovial fluid are fat globules. CPPD crystals are sometimes better visualized with ordinary light than with compensated polarized light because they may be very weakly birefringent under polarized light. (b) The microscopic field in (a), viewed under compensated polarized light microscopy, x 400. Note the prominent rhomboid-shaped intracellular crystal in the upper center portion of the photograph. Reproduced with permission from Schumacher HR, Reginato AJ. *Atlas of Synovial Fluid Analysis and Crystal Identification*. Philadelphia: Lea & Febiger, 1991

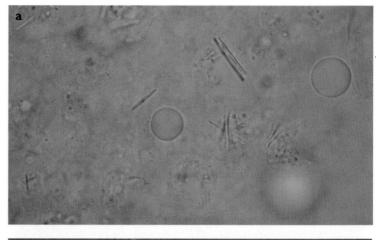

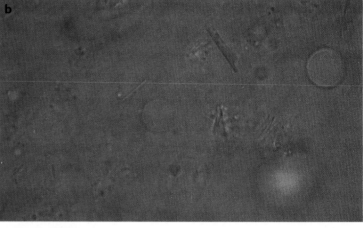

Figure 5 (a) Pleomorphic clumps of calcium hydroxyapatite crystals in synovial fluid from a patient with osteoarthritis. Wet preparation, viewed under ordinary light, x100. (b) Alizarin red stain of the same fluid, wet preparation x10. The clumps of apatite stain strongly. Reproduced with permission from Schumacher HR, Reginato AJ. *Atlas of Synovial Fluid Analysis and Crystal Identification*. Philadelphia: Lea & Febiger, 1991

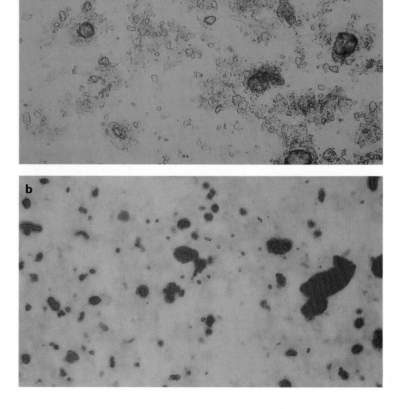

Figure 6 Large, plate-shaped crystals with notched corners, characteristic of cholesterol monohydrate. Cholesterol crystals are common in chronic effusions of joints and bursae of patients with rheumatoid arthritis and, occasionally, are present in the synovial fluid of patients with osteoarthritis. Compensated polarized light, x400. Reproduced with permission from Schumacher HR, Reginato AJ. *Atlas of Synovial Fluid Analysis and Crystal Identification*. Philadelphia: Lea & Febiger, 1991

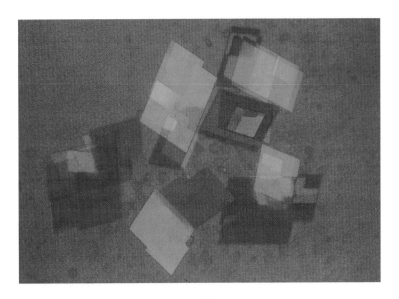

Figure 7 Gram stain of synovial fluid from a patient with osteoarthritis who acquired an acute bacterial joint infection. Note the numerous polymorphonuclear leukocytes and abundant Gram-positive cocci, many of which are in chains. Cultures grew *Streptococcus pneumoniae*

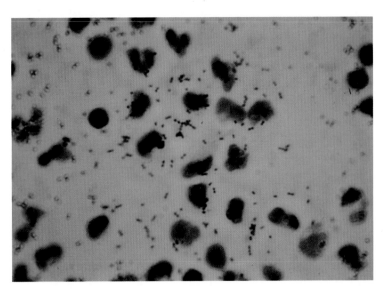

Figure 8 LE cell in synovial fluid aspirated from the knee of a 70-year-old male with a classic history and X-ray findings of osteoarthritis, who also had drug-induced systemic lupus erythematosus associated with the use of procainamide for cardiac arrhythmias. In addition to the development of knee effusions, the patient had mild leucopenia and thrombocytopenia. Photograph kindly provided by M. Benson, MD

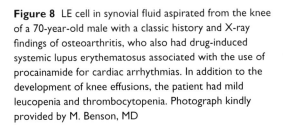

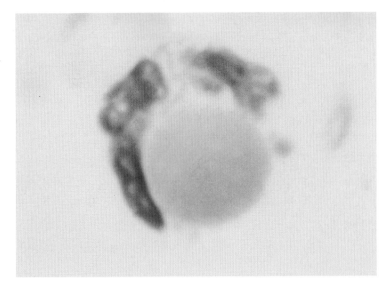

Figure 9 Talc crystals in synovial fluid. These are strongly positively birefringent and can be recognized by their shape, which often is not completely round. Magnification x2000, original magnification, x400. From Krey PR, Lazaro DM. Analysis of Synovial Fluid. In Brandt KD, ed. *Diagnostic Studies in Rheumatology.* Summit, NJ: Ciba-Geigy Corporation, 1992

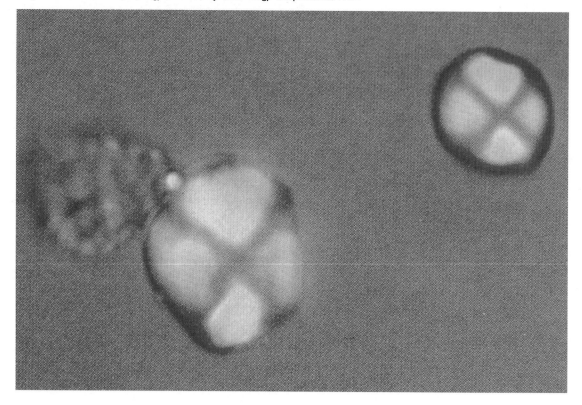

References

1 Krey PR, Lazaro DM. Analysis of synovial fluid. In Brandt KD, ed. *Diagnostic Studies in Rheumatology.* Summit, NJ: Ciba-Geigy Corporation, 1992

2 Ropes MW, Bauer W. *Synovial Fluid Changes in Joint Disease.* Cambridge, MA: Harvard University Press, 1953

3 Krey PR, Bailen DA. Synovial fluid leukocytosis: a study of extremes. *Am J Med* 1979;67:436–42

4 Cohen AS, Brandt KD, Krey PR. Synovial fluid. In Cohen AS, ed. *Laboratory Diagnostic Procedures in the Rheumatoid Diseases,* 2nd edn. Boston, MA: Little, Brown, 1975:1–62

5 Schumacher HR, Reginato AJ. *Atlas of Synovial Fluid and Crystal Identification.* Philadelphia: Lea & Febiger, 1991

CHAPTER EIGHT
Radiography of osteoarthritis

The diagnosis of osteoarthritis (OA) is usually based on clinical and radiographic features. In the early stages of the disease X-rays may be normal but, as articular cartilage is lost, narrowing of the inter-bone distance becomes evident (Figures 1, 2 and 3). Other characteristic X-ray findings include sub-chondral cysts, subchondral sclerosis and marginal osteophytes, which represent the response of the bone to the increased mechanical load resulting from cartilage degeneration (Figures 2 and 3). A sub-set of OA, erosive OA (EOA), involves the distal and proximal interphalangeal joints and is marked by more pain and tenderness and soft tissue swelling than generally seen in typical nodal OA. Bone erosion, with collapse of the subchondral plate, is common in patients with knee EOA, in whom the changes may proceed to bony ankylosis. While the clinical signs of inflammation may be so marked as to resemble rheumatoid arthritis, this form of OA is limited to the finger joints (Figure 4). Although some investigators have suggested that the primary abnormality in OA is in the bone and that the changes in the overlying cartilage are secondary, this represents a minority opinion.

Disparity between the severity of radiographic findings and severity of symptoms or functional impairment in subjects with OA is common. While some X-ray evidence of OA in weight-bearing joints is present in more than 90% of people over the age of 40, only about 30% will have symptoms. For example, among men with advanced X-ray changes of hip OA, e.g. as depicted in Figure 5, nearly 50% may not have joint pain (Figure 6). As noted in the chapter on Epidemiology, risk factors for pain and disability in OA are different from those related to joint pathology.

Figure 1 Osteoarthritis of the knee. Note the narrowing of the medial tibiofemoral joint space bilaterally. This is generally considered to be due to loss of articular cartilage, although 'false positives' are common. For example, a minor degree of knee flexion can result in significant narrowing of the tibiofemoral joint space. Small osteophytes are present on the medial border of the medial tibial plateau in both knees

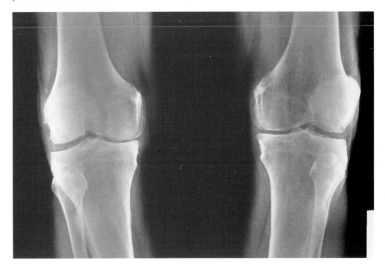

Figure 2 Bilateral hip osteoarthritis. Note narrowing of the joint space in the superolateral pole of each hip, subchondral sclerosis and osteophytosis on both the acetabular and femoral components of the joint. Subchondral cysts are also apparent

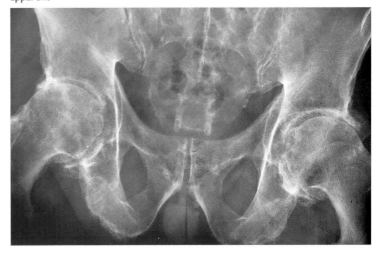

Figure 3 OA of the elbow. (a) Lateral radiograph. Note the narrowing of the inter-bone distance in the radiohumeral joint, the subchondral sclerosis and the osteophytic peaking of both the distal humerus and the ulna. (b) Anteroposterior view shows prominent osteophytes at the humeral and ulnar margins of the joint (arrows)

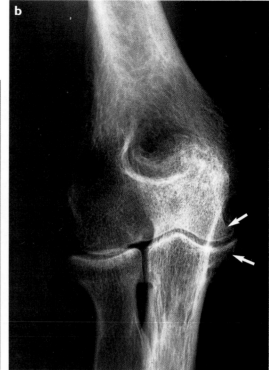

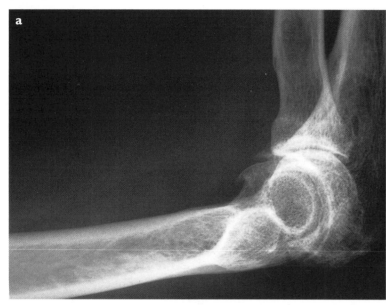

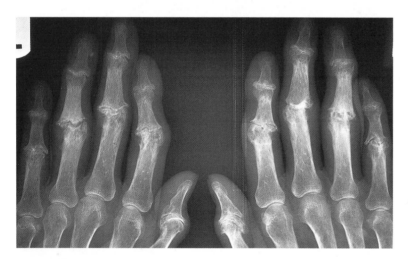

Figure 4 Erosive osteoarthritis. Note the marked deformity of the proximal interphalangeal joint of the left long finger and, in particular, the collapse of the subchondral plate, due to bony destruction, which is obvious in several inter-phalangeal joints. The joint disease in this form of OA may progress to bony ankylosis

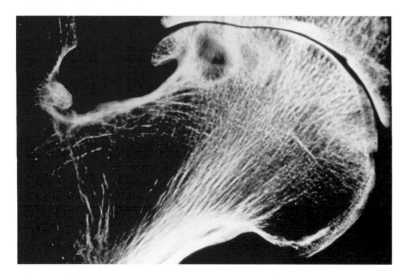

Figure 5 Radiograph of the hip of a patient with advanced osteoarthritis. Note the extensive loss of articular cartilage, reflected by marked narrowing of the joint space; bony sclerosis, with thickening of the subchondral plate; large subchondral cyst on the superolateral aspect of the femoral head; and the prominent osteophytes on the acetabulum and the femoral head

Table I Kellgren and Lawrence grading criteria for radiographic severity of knee osteoarthritis

Grade	OA severity	Radiographic findings
0	None	No features of OA
I	Doubtful	Minute osteophyte, doubtful significance
II	Minimal	Definite osteophyte, unimpaired joint space
III	Moderate	Moderate diminution of joint space
IV	Severe	Joint space greatly impaired, with sclerosis of subchondral bone

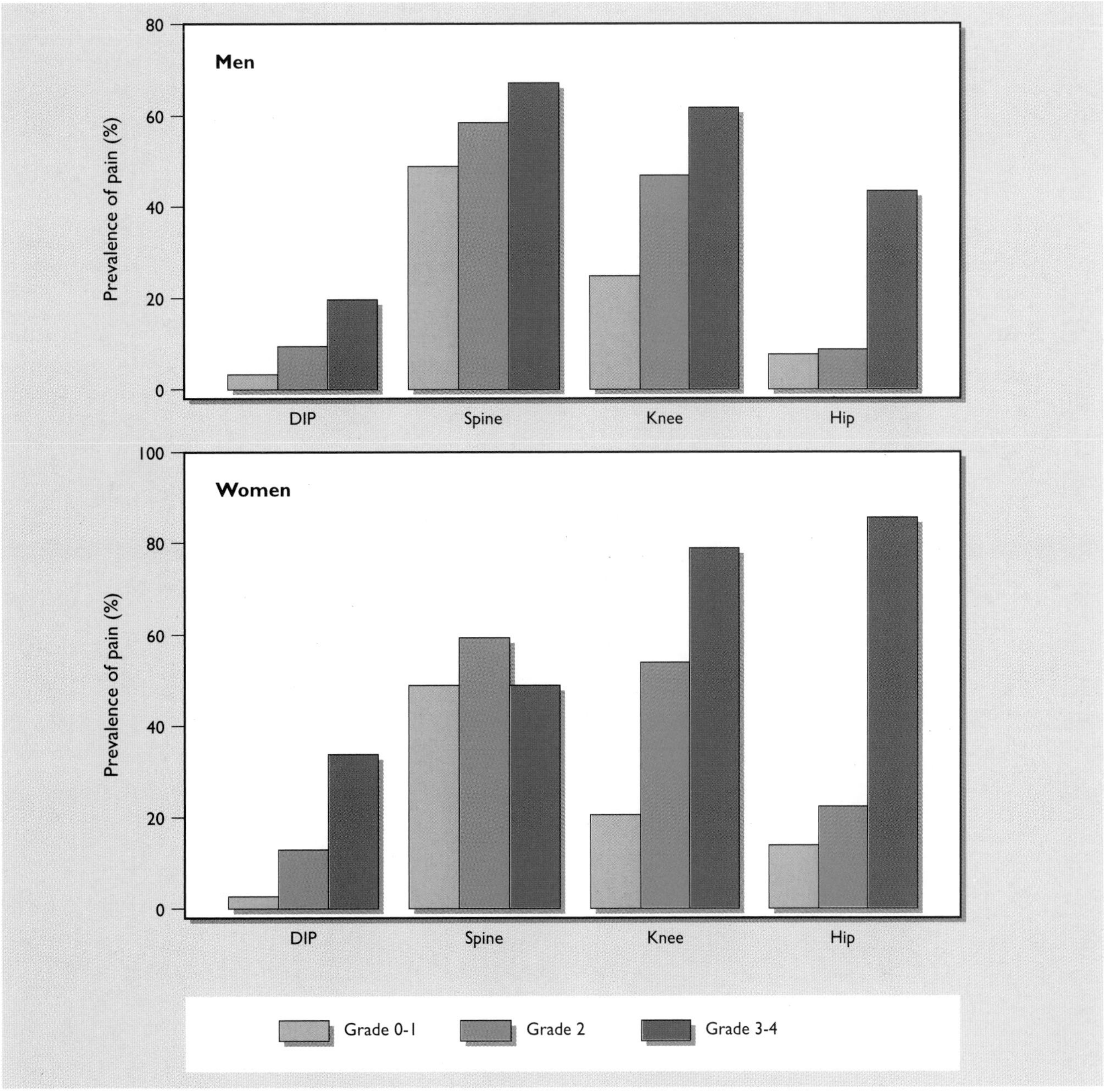

Figure 6 The prevalence of pain at various joint sites in relationship to the radiographic severity of OA, based on the Kellgren and Lawrence (K&L) grade. DIP, distal interphalangeal joint. From O'Reilly S, Doherty M. Clinical features of osteoarthritis and standard approaches to the diagnosis. Signs, symptoms, and laboratory tests. In Brandt KD, Lohmander S, Doherty M, eds. *Osteoarthritis.* Oxford: Oxford University Press, 1998:197–217

From Kellgren JH, Lawrence JS. Radiologic assessment of osteoarthritis. *Ann Rheum Dis* 1957;16:494–501; and The Department of Rheumatology and Medical Illustration, University of Manchester. *The Epidemiology of Chronic Rheumatism. Atlas of Standard Radiographs of Arthritis.* Philadelphia: FA Davis Company, 1973;2:1–15

Men

Prevalence of pain (%)

DIP   Spine   Knee   Hip

Women

Prevalence of pain (%)

DIP   Spine   Knee   Hip

Grade 0-1   Grade 2   Grade 3-4

Figure 7 K&L grading of radiographic severity of OA. (a) Normal knee radiograph, K&L Grade 0; (b) mild but definite osteophyte formation, with essentially normal joint space width, K&L Grade II; (c) osteophytosis with marked narrowing of the joint space in the medial tibiofemoral compartment, K&L Grade III; (d) complete loss of joint space in the medial tibiofemoral compartment, with prominent osteophytes and subchondral sclerosis of the medial tibial plateau, K&L Grade IV

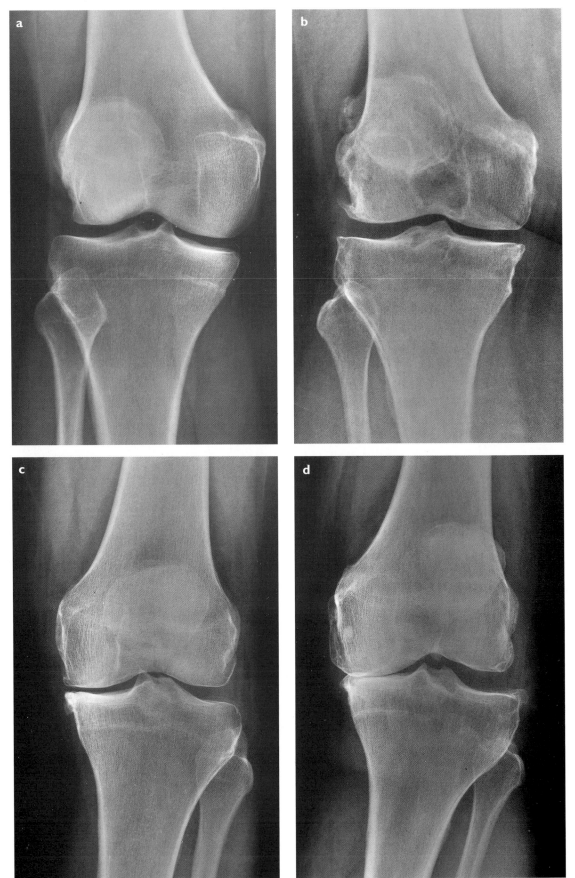

Figure 8 Patient with typical clinical features of knee OA, i.e. pain in both knees aggravated by weight bearing and relieved by rest, with bony crepitus bilaterally. A definite osteophyte is present on the medial tibial plateau of the left knee. The right knee shows no X-ray evidence of osteophytes but prominent subchondral sclerosis of the medial tibial plateau and some mild narrowing of the medial tibiofemoral joint space, emphasizing that the severity of individual radiographic features of OA in a given joint may be highly discordant

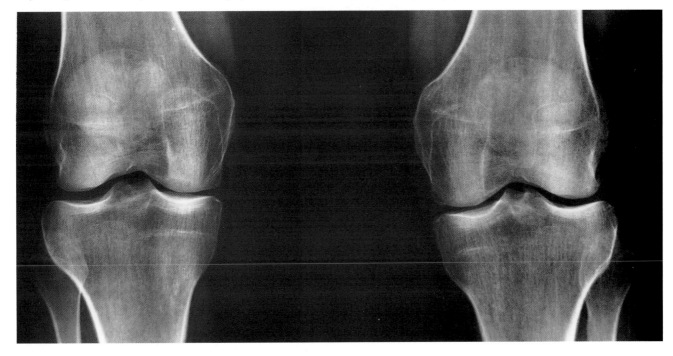

Figure 9 Conventional knee radiography. (a) Standing anteroposterior view of the knee in full extension, illustrating poor centering of the tibial spines under the femoral notch and poor alignment of the central X-ray beam with the medial tibial plateau, reflected by the lack of superimposition of the anterior and posterior margins of the medial tibial plateau (arrows). (b) Semiflexed anteroposterior view of the knee depicted in (a), with optimal fluoroscopic positioning of the knee providing flexion of the joint, superimposing the anterior and posterior margins of the medial plateau (arrow), and rotation of the foot, centering the tibial spines under the femoral notch. Reproduced with permission from Mazzuca S, Brandt KD. Osteoarthritis. Plain radiography as an outcome measure in clinical trials of OA. In Brandt KD, ed. *Rheum Dis Clin N Amer* Philadelphia: WB Saunders Co., 1999:467–80

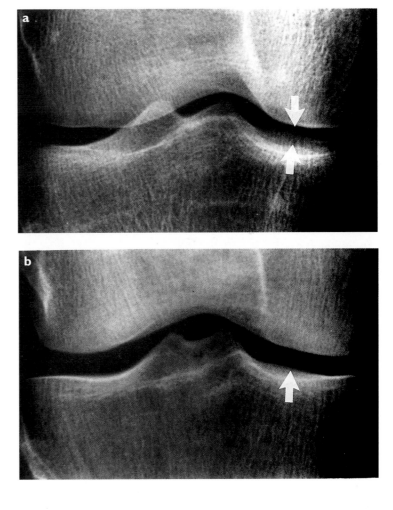

Figure 10 Sample size and duration of hypothetical clinical trials of a disease-modifying osteoarthritis drug in which medial tibiofemoral joint space width is measured with a standard error of measurement (SE_m) reflecting uniformly poor technical quality (0.40 mm), intermediate quality (0.31 mm), or uniformly high quality (0.25 mm). The upper panel depicts differences in the sample size which would be required for a 24-month trial under each of the above conditions, assuming that the drug being tested retards joint space narrowing by 30%, relative to the placebo. The lower panel depicts differences in the duration of treatment required if the sample size were 200 knees per treatment group in each condition. Reproduced with permission from Mazzuca S, Brandt KD. Osteoarthritis. Plain radiography as an outcome measure in clinical trials of OA. In Brandt KD, ed. *Rheum Dis Clin N Amer.* Philadelphia: WB Saunders Co., 1999:467–80

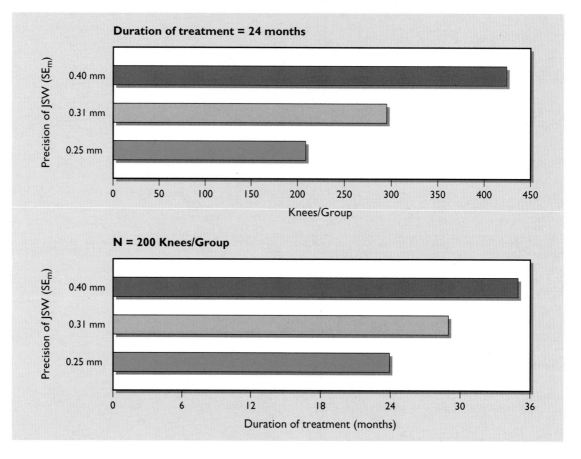

A knee X-ray taken while the subject is standing is more likely to exhibit joint space narrowing – the surrogate of articular cartilage thinning – than one obtained in the supine position. However, when we examined the relationship between articular cartilage degeneration and joint space narrowing in standing anteroposterior knee radiographs of patients with chronic knee pain, most of whom had X-ray findings of only mild OA, we found 33% of those with tibiofemoral joint space narrowing had grossly normal cartilage at arthroscopy, i.e. they had a 'false-positive' radiograph. Joint space narrowing in these patients with chronic knee pain and relatively mild X-ray changes of OA did not predict the status of the articular cartilage. Although it remains the 'gold standard' for assessing the progression of OA, the conventional standing knee radiograph is not a sensitive technique for identifying articular cartilage changes in OA.

As pointed out by Buckland-Wright, the steps required to obtained a standard radiograph make quality control difficult:

1 The clinician making the request may not indicate precisely what is required (images of many OA knees are still obtained with the subject lying down).

2 The technician may have his or her own idiosyncratic methods of positioning patients, especially when faced with someone who has difficulty standing or walking.

3 The person evaluating the X-ray may be unaware of what has gone on beforehand. In addition to the variability in the skill of the technician, variability within the radiologic and mensural processes can lead to errors in assessment of the dimensions of various features recorded in the radiograph.

4 When a standing knee X-ray is obtained, the positioning of the subject is extremely important. Minor degrees of flexion may result in significant joint space narrowing.

To cite one example of the difficulties in obtaining an optimal image: although radiographic magnification is not generally taken into account, it will be affected by the distance between the center of the joint and the film. This distance will, in turn, be affected by both the size and the positioning of the patient. Therefore, it will be influenced by obesity and by restriction of joint movement due to pain or buttressing osteophytes. In imaging of the hip this usually does not present much of a problem but it is particularly relevant to knee radiography because most patients with knee OA are obese. Magnification in a knee X-ray can be as great as 35%. The common practice of assuming that magnification of the image of large joints is x1.0 leads to inaccurate measurement of joint space width.

The grading scale which has been employed most widely for assessment of the severity of OA, the Kellgren and Lawrence (K&L) scale (Table 1, Figure 7), was developed before the demonstration that the standing knee X-ray is more sensitive for the assessment of joint space narrowing than a radiograph taken with the patient supine. It permits a diagnosis of definite OA in the presence of osteophytosis alone, i.e. in the absence of joint space narrowing. As indicated above, however, loss of articular cartilage, not osteophytosis, is the predominant pathologic feature of OA. Indeed, in the absence of joint space narrowing or other bony changes, osteophytosis may be due to aging and not to OA.

Furthermore, all semi-quantitative scoring systems, including the K&L scale, suffer from two limitations, which are based on the following assumptions: (1) that the change in any radiographic feature (e.g. joint spacing narrowing, osteophytes) is linear and constant during the course of the disease and (2) that the relationship between the different radiographic features of OA is constant. Neither of these assumptions is valid. In most cases the rate of progression of X-ray severity is not constant but advances in a step-wise fashion; and the individual radiographic features of OA do not progress at comparable rates. In some patients, for example, the rate of joint space loss may be much greater than the rate of osteophyte growth, or vice versa (Figure 8). The essential point is that neither osteophytosis nor joint space narrowing provides an accurate assessment of the intra-articular pathology in patients with relatively early OA.

Alternative approaches for the detection of early OA, such as scintigraphy, ultrasonography and magnetic resonance imaging, are under study. Conventional radiography, performed with standardization of positioning of the joint (usually by fluoroscopy), coupled with computerized measurement of joint space width on the digitized image, although not practical (or necessary) for routine clinical care, may have great utility in clinical trials aimed at determining whether a drug can slow the rate of joint damage in OA (Figure 9). This approach has been shown to afford much greater reproducibility in the measurement of joint space width than the conventional standing extended view knee X-ray (coefficient of variation for repeated measures = approximately 5% vs 20%). Use of this highly standardized methodology in a clinical trial of a drug which may modify structural damage of the joint can provide an important advantage: the duration of the trial can be shorter, or the number of subjects needed to demonstrate a significant drug effect smaller, than in a study in which radiography is less reproducible (Figure 10).

While serial radiography may be essential in a clinical trial evaluating a drug or biological agent for its potential to modify structural damage in OA, in clinical practice serial X-rays of the patient with OA are seldom indicated. At the initial clinic visit it is reasonable to obtain an X-ray of the joint involved to assess the degree of pathology and exclude other causes of the patient's joint pain (e.g. rheumatoid disease, crystal deposition disease, infection), but repeat X-rays of the OA joint are generally not necessary unless the patient becomes a candidate for joint surgery or the rate of progression of the disease accelerates markedly.

Bibliography

Buckland-Wright JC. Quantitation of radiographic changes. In Brandt KD, Lohmander S, Doherty M, eds. *Osteoarthritis*. Oxford: Oxford University Press, 1998:459–72

Department of Rheumatology and Medical Illustration, University of Manchester. *The Epidemiology of Chronic Rheumatism. Atlas of Standard Radiographs of Arthritis*. Philadelphia: FA Davis Company, 1973;2:1–15

Fife RS, Brandt KD, Braunstein EM, *et al*. Relationship between arthroscopic evidence of cartilage damage and radiographic evidence of joint space narrowing in early osteoarthritis of the knee. *Arthritis Rheum* 1991;34:377–82

Kellgren JH, Lawrence JS. Radiologic assessment of osteoarthritis. *Ann Rheum Dis* 1957;16:494–501

Lawrence JS, Bremmer JM, Bier F. Osteoarthrosis: prevalence in the population and relationship between symptoms and X-ray changes. *Ann Rheum Dis* 1966;25:1–23

Mazzuca S, Brandt KD. Plain radiography as an outcome measure in clinical trials of OA. In Brandt KD, ed. *Rheumatic Disease Clinics of North America. Osteoarthritis*. Philadelphia: WB Saunders Co, 1999:467–80

CHAPTER NINE

Monitoring the patient with osteoarthritis

The basic goals in managing osteoarthritis are to reduce symptoms (pain, stiffness, instability) and maintain or improve function. Accordingly, it is important to be able to determine whether the patient is getting better or worse. In advanced disease, when significant structural damage is present, the assessment of pain in weight-bearing joints is confounded by the fact that the patient adapts to his pain by avoiding activities which aggravate symptoms. These self-imposed limitations further aggravate the problem by accelerating physical deconditioning.

Monitoring of the patient with osteoarthritis over time should include periodic global rating by the physician and the patient, a simple pain assessment, a count of flares, an assessment of function, a focused examination and selective performance testing (Table 1). Although X-ray imaging may be important to confirm the diagnosis, because it correlates poorly with symptoms and function it has little value in the routine monitoring of patients. A repeat X-ray is needed only when surgery is under consideration or when a major change in symptoms or physical findings has occurred.

Definitions

Impairment, disability and handicap are the major ways in which an illness impacts on an individual.

Impairment is an objective loss of psychologic, physiologic, or anatomic structure or function and signifies a pathological state. In OA, impairment may be measured radiographically (for example by

Table I Items related to pain and stiffness in outcome instruments which may be used to monitor patients with hip or knee osteoarthritis

Variables	Disease and joint-specific		Arthritis-specific		Generic		
	WOMAC	Lequesne	AIMS	HAQ	SF-36	NHP	SIP
Pain							
General			•	•	•	•	•
Sitting or lying	•	•					•
Night	•	•					•
Standing	•	•					
Walking	•	•					•
Negotiating stairs	•						
Medication(s)							
Stiffness							
Morning	•	•	•				
After resting	•						

WOMAC, Western Ontario and McMaster Universities OA Index; HAQ, Health Assessment Questionnaire; Lequesne, Algofunctional indices for hip and knee; AIMS, Arthritis Impact Measurement scale; SF-36, MOS-Short Form 36; NHP, Nottingham Health Profile; SIP, Sickness Impact Profile

Figure 1 Clinical assessment of the patient with osteoarthritis. Three evaluations may be performed at the initial visit and then at 6-month intervals

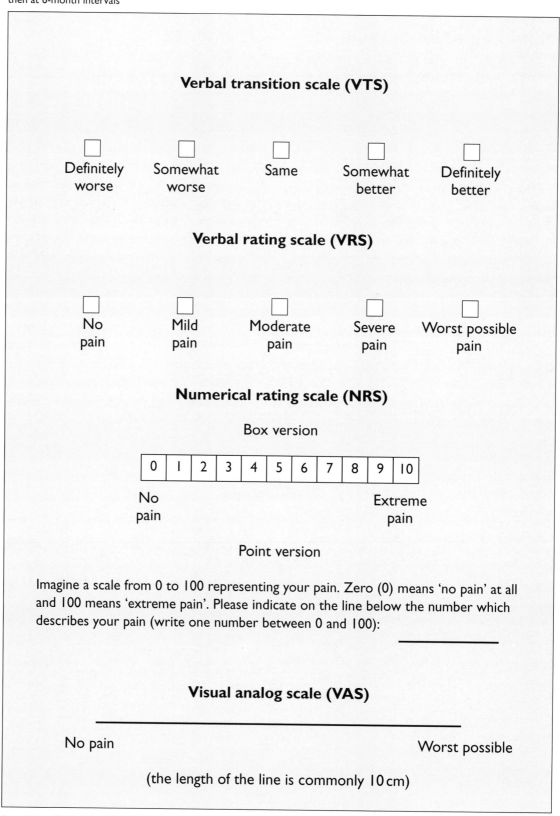

From Bellamy N. Methods of clinical assessment of anti-rheumatic drugs. Baillière's *Clin Rheumatol* 1988;2:339–62

assessment of articular cartilage thickness) or clinically (e.g. by assessment of joint deformity and range of motion).

Disability in the performance of normal activities can arise as the result of an impairment. Disability, in turn, can affect behavior, communication, personal care, locomotion, dexterity and the performance of activities of daily living. At any given time disability is determined by three factors: capacity, will and need. 'Capacity' is the physical and mental ability to do something. 'Will' includes personality factors, such as drive and motivation. 'Need' refers to the necessity for the patient to perform a function. In clinical practice, function may be improved by enhancing capacity, will or need.

Handicap is the disadvantage for an individual that limits fulfillment of normal function. Handicaps include work ability, social integration and economic self-sufficiency.

Symptoms of functional difficulties due to OA should be considered in the context of the patient's experience. While some clinicians hold the view that, because it is subjective, the patient's report is less important than hard, objective, clinical findings, studies show that patient-derived data are reliable, valid and as sensitive as – or more sensitive than – traditional radiographic measurements or physical findings.

Pain scales

Pain may be evaluated during an office visit by a verbal transition scale (VTS), a verbal rating scale (VRS), a numerical rating scale (NRS) or a visual analog scale (VAS) (Figure 1). The VTS asks the patient to estimate whether the pain has been stable or has changed over a period of time (for better or worse). The VRS asks the patient to quantify his pain, for example from total absence of pain to extreme pain, with a number of intermediate levels (mild, moderate, severe). The NRS asks the patient to assign a number from an ordinal scale, usually ranging from 0 (no pain) to 10 (extreme pain), or from 0 to 100, rather than asking him to choose an adjective. The VAS typically employs a 10-cm line on which the patient marks a point representing his level of pain. The distance from this point to the origin of the line is then recorded. All of these

techniques show changes when a therapeutic intervention is effective.

Health status or quality of life instruments

A variety of self-administered or interviewer-assisted instruments may be used to evaluate and monitor the patient with OA. Generic measures have been developed for general populations. Others are disease-specific or organ-specific (Tables 1, 2 and 3). These may be administered to the patient on an office visit while he is waiting to be seen by the physician.

Measurement of general health status, or quality of life, is used to assess broadly the patient's overall state as it is influenced by physical, emotional and social functioning. The MOS Short 36-Item Form (SF-36), the most widely used generic health status measure, is a self-administered questionnaire which takes less than 10 minutes to complete. It has excellent psychometric properties and has been validated and tested for reliability in OA. Other generic health status questionnaires which may be used in patients with OA include the Sickness Impact Profile (SIP) and Nottingham Health Profile (NHP).

In contrast to the general health status measures, the Lequesne Indexes of Severity for Osteoarthritis of the hip and the knee and the Western Ontario and McMaster Universities Osteoarthritis Index (WOMAC) are disease- and joint-specific instruments which were designed for OA patients.

The Lequesne Indexes consist of one 10-item scale for the knee and another 10-item scale for the hip. Either can be administered by a trained individual in 5–10 minutes. Both rate pain or discomfort, stiffness, performance of the activities of daily living, and the need for an assistive device to achieve maximum walking capacity. In the hip scale an additional question addresses arthritis-related sexual dysfunction in sexually active women.

The WOMAC is a single 24-item questionnaire focusing on pain, stiffness and functional limitations related to knee and/or hip OA. It is available in two essentially equivalent versions, one using a VRS and another using a VAS. Both versions are self-reported and can be completed in less than 5 minutes. The VRS version can be administered by

Table 2 Items related to physical function in outcome instruments which may be used to monitor patients with hip or knee osteoarthritis

Variables	Disease and joint-specific		Arthritis-specific		Generic		
	WOMAC	Lequesne	AIMS	HAQ	SF-36	NHP	SIP
Physical function							
Standing	•					•	•
Sitting	•						
Lying	•						•
Squatting or bending knee		•			•		•
Bending to the floor	•	•		•	•	•	•
Walking on flat ground	•	•	•	•	•	•	•
Walking on uneven ground		•					
Walking aids		•	•	•		•	•
Stair climbing going up	•	•	•	•	•	•	•
going down	•	•					•
Transfers bed	•			•		•	•
chair				•		•	•
toilet	•		•	•			•
bath tub	•		•	•		•	•
car	•	•		•			•
public transportation			•				•
Dressing general			•	•	•		•
putting on socks/stockings	•	•				•	•
Domestic duties light work	•		•	•	•	•	•
heavy work	•		•	•	•	•	•
shopping	•		•	•	•		•
Sexual activity		•	•			•	•

WOMAC, Western Ontario and McMaster Universities OA Index; HAQ, Health Assessment Questionnaire; Lequesne, Algofunctional indices for hip and knee; AIMS, Arthritis Impact Measurement Scale; SF-36, MOS-Short Form 36; NHP, Nottingham Health Profile; SIP, Sickness Impact Profile

Table 3 Items related to mental health in outcome instruments which may be used to monitor patients with hip or knee osteoarthritis

Variables	Disease and joint-specific		Arthritis-specific		Generic		
	WOMAC	Lequesne	AIMS	HAQ	SF-36	NHP	SIP
Mental health							
Communication			•		•	•	•
Social life			•		•	•	•
Leisure activities				•	•	•	
Mood			•		•	•	•

WOMAC, Western Ontario and McMaster Universities OA Index; HAQ, Health Assessment Questionnaire; Lequesne, Algofunctional indices for hip and knee; AIMS, Arthritis Impact Measurement Scale; SF-36, MOS-Short Form 36; NHP, Nottingham Health Profile; SIP, Sickness Impact Profile

telephone. The WOMAC has been extensively tested for validity, reliability and responsiveness and has been used as a main outcome measure in evaluations of drugs, surgery and acupuncture.

While the Lequesne Indexes and the WOMAC have the advantage of being OA-specific, two other instruments, which are arthritis-specific but not disease-specific, also enjoy popularity and may be useful for serial evaluation of the OA patient on office visits. These are the Arthritis Impact Measurement scale (AIMS) and Health Assessment Questionnaire (HAQ).

Quantitative approaches applied to the practice setting

Table 4 summarizes the components of a comprehensive and practical assessment of the OA patient which takes into account the practical limitations of routine office care. The approach, which can be employed at the initial visit and at regular intervals thereafter (e.g. every 6 months), follows a step-wise progression, beginning with traditional open-ended screening questions which can rapidly establish the patient's priorities and assess whether the condition has changed. If deterioration has occurred, the questions progress to a more detailed inquiry and

systematic review. Observation of the patient's gait and ability to transfer from a chair and to the examination table will confirm reported problems and facilitate the physician's assessment of his patient's status relative to that of other patients with the same impairments.

When the patient reports a change in his problems, additional history, particularly details of medication use and changes in activity, may provide insight into potential management strategies. When severe discomfort is reported, knowing which critical functions are disturbed (e.g. sleep, weight bearing) will assist the physician in interpreting the impact of the patient's pain. Physical examination can identify coexisting periarticular soft tissue rheumatism (trochanteric, iliopsoas or anserine bursitis; supraspinatus tendinitis; nerve entrapment syndrome) which may respond to local therapy. Biomechanical factors, such as flexion deformities, recurvatum and valgus or varus deformities, which may cause ligament strain, can be managed with orthoses or surgery. Finally, determination of whether putting the joint through its full range of motion produces discomfort may provide insight into unreported functional limitations. For

Table 4 Clinical assessment of the patient with osteoarthritis to be performed initially and at 6-month intervals thereafter

Variables	Assessment
Global rating	Verbal transition scale: *Are you better, same or worse?*

Pain	Numerical scale: *Over the last month, how much discomfort have you had on a scale of 1–5 (5 is the most)?*
	Have you had:
	    Pain at rest?
	    Pain with any weight bearing?
	    Pain at night?

Function	*What is the most difficult thing for you to do on a regular day?*
Flares	Number of exacerbations or joint effusions?
Examination	Range of motion and effect of movement on pain Functional testing, if necessary (see Table 5)
Therapy	Analgesics NSAIDs Joint aspirations Intra-articular steroid injections

Joint effusion, accumulation of joint fluid, documented by a physician; NSAIDs, nonsteroidal anti-inflammatory drugs

Table 5 Screening for functional disability in the patient with osteoarthritis

Task	Musculoskeletal area tested	Function
Touch fingers to palmar crease[†]	Finger small joints (F)	Grip
Touch index finger pad to thumb pad	Thumb joints, (AB, O) and thumb opponens muscle (S)	Grip and pinch
Place palm of hand to contralateral trochanter	Wrist (F) and shoulder (AD)	Hygiene (perineal and back care)
Touch 1st MCP joint to top of head	Shoulder (AB, F, ER) and elbow (F)	Hygiene (face, neck, hair, oral), feeding and dressing
Touch waist in back	Shoulder (IR)	Dressing and low back care
Touch tip of shoe	Back, hip and knee (F) and elbow (E)	Dressing of lower extremities
Arise from chair without using hands[‡]	Hip girdle and quadriceps rectus femoris (S)	Transfer ability
Stand unassisted	Hip, knee and ankle (F, E) and quadriceps femoris muscle (S)	Standing
Step over a 6-inch block	Hip, knee, ankle (F, E) and hip girdle (S)	Stairs
Gait	Hip, knee, ankle and small joints of feet (F, E), hip girdle and quadriceps femoris muscle (S)	Walking

AB, abduction; ER, external rotation; F, flexion; E, extension; AD, adduction; IR, internal rotation; O, opposition; S, strength; [†]if abnormal, test grip strength; [‡] if abnormal, test ability to get up from bed. Adapted from Liang MH, Gall V, Partridge AJ, Eaton H. Management of functional disability in homebound patients. *J Fam Pract* 1983;17:429–35

the unreliable historian, a simple performance test (Table 5) is a quick way to identify potential functional problems and the joints involved.

Rating of pain by the patient and physician

Patients may be asked to rate their symptoms over a defined period of time (e.g. a week, a month, since their last visit) using a VRS, NRS or TRS (Figure 1). The physician might rate pain lower than expected for patients with a high threshold or those taking pain medication, or higher than expected for patients with a low threshold or nonorganic pain. The physician's perception of the patient's pain can be substantiated by examination and observation of the patient's behavior. Spontaneous attempts by the patient to avoid a painful activity or painful examination and facial expressions of discomfort can be used to develop a clinical grading scale, such as:

0 = no spontaneous complaint;

1 = spontaneous complaint;

2 = wincing only with movement;

3 = wincing and withdrawal with movement; and

4 = wincing with activity and the presence of night pain.

Evaluation of function

It is important to recognize the natural trajectory of functional decline which is accelerated by chronic and acute illness in the patient with OA. Many individuals decline slowly, accommodate to their decline in function, and accept their limitations. Because, by the time function has declined, effective intervention may be difficult, regular periodic functional evaluation is important. Function is an important endpoint and should be assessed in a standardized, quantitative manner. Two approaches may be employed: a 1-second drill asks the patient what single function is the most difficult for him or her to perform during the day and how difficult it is on a scale of 1 to 5; a 10-second drill enables the

Table 6 A 10-second inventory of function for use with the patient with osteoarthritis

How does your condition affect you?

What is the most:

(1) difficult thing for you to do in an average day?

(2) important thing for us to work on?

What can't you do:

(1) that you were able to do?

(2) that you need or would like to do?

Are you able to sleep through the night?

patient to express how he is affected by the condition, to communicate which activity is the most difficult, to compare his condition to baseline, and to determine priority for treatment (Table 6). In patients with polyarticular OA, or when the patient is a poor observer or cognitively impaired, an inventory may be taken of activities of daily living (ADL), such as **a**mbulation, **d**ressing, **e**ating, **p**ersonal hygiene, **t**ransfers, and **t**oileting (The acronym ADEPTT provides a mnemonic aid). In addition, one of the disease-specific or joint-specific instruments (Tables 2–4) may be administered while the patient is waiting to be seen by the physician. The visit can then incorporate and amplify the results obtained by means of the questionnaire.

Performance testing provides a useful method of evaluating function in elderly, sick, cognitively impaired or unreliable subjects. A rapid office test which is useful in screening for potential problems has the patient imitate the examiner in the performance of maneuvers that test musculoskeletal areas (Table 5). If the patient is unable to perform these maneuvers or they cause pain, or if asymmetry exists between sides, limitations in certain self-care areas are likely.

Bibliography

Bellamy N, Buchanan WW, Goldsmith CH, *et al.* Validation study of WOMAC: a health status instrument for measuring clinically important patient relevant outcomes to antirheumatic drug therapy in patients with osteoarthritis of the hip or knee. *J Rheumatol* 1988;15:1833–40

Bergner M, Bobbitt RA, Pollard WE, *et al.* The Sickness Impact Profile: validation of a health status measure. *Med Care* 1976;14:57–67

Lequesne MG, Mery C, Samson M, Gerard P. Indexes of severity for osteoarthritis of the hip and knee. Validation – value in comparison with other assessment tests. *Scand J Rheumatol* (Suppl) 1987;65:85–9

Liang MH, Jette AM. Measuring functional ability in chronic arthritis: a critical review. *Arthritis Rheum* 1981;24:80–6

Meenan RF, Gertman PM, Mason JH. Measuring health status in arthritis. The arthritis impact measurement scales. *Arthritis Rheum* 1980;23:146–52

Pincus T, Summey JA, Soraci SA Jr, *et al.* Assessment of patient satisfaction in activities of daily living using a modified Stanford Health Assessment Questionnaire. *Arthritis Rheum* 1983;26:1346–53

Rivest C, Liang MH. Evaluating outcome in osteoarthritis for research and clinical practice. *Osteoarthritis.* Brandt KD, Doherty M, Lohmander SL, eds. Oxford: Oxford University Press, 1998:403–14

Ware JE Jr, Sherbourne CD. The MOS 36-item short-form health survey (SF-36). A conceptual framework and item selection. *Med Care* 1992;30:473–83

SECTION THREE

Therapy

CHAPTER 10

Nonmedicinal therapy for osteoarthritis pain

Exercise

The current approach of most physicians to management of osteoarthritis (OA) today is aimed at reducing joint pain through pharmacologic measures. To a much lesser extent than drugs, range of motion (ROM) exercises and muscle strengthening exercises are prescribed for patients with OA. Unfortunately, these exercises generally focus only on the impairment (muscle weakness, loss of motion, pain) in and around the involved joint. However, because OA can result in severe functional limitation and disability, effective management requires more than attention only to the localized impairment; the prescribed exercise regimen must also address functional limitations and disability arising secondary to inactivity. As noted by Minor, goals of an exercise program for the patient with OA should be:

1 reduction of impairment and improvement of function; i.e. reduction of joint pain, increases in ROM and strength, normalization of gait and facilitation of the performance of daily activities;

2 protection of the OA joint from further damage by reducing stress on the joint, attenuating joint forces, and improving biomechanics;

3 prevention of disability and poor health secondary to inactivity by increasing the daily level of physical activity and improving physical fitness.

The exercise program for the patient with OA should be individualized. In the patient with significant weakness or reduction in joint motion, the initial aim should be to reduce the impairment, improve function and prepare for increased activity. For the patient in whom strength and ROM are reasonably good, the exercise program should focus on joint protection strategies and general conditioning.

For knee OA, a combination of exercises, including ROM, strengthening and low impact aerobic exercise, is appropriate. However, two precautions should be considered before implementation of an exercise program in patients with OA. First, exercise of an acutely inflamed or significantly swollen joint should be deferred until the acute inflammation has subsided. Second, before initiation of an aerobic exercise program, an exercise stress test should be performed to identify cardiac disease; the objective of the proposed aerobic program should be to achieve 60–80% of the target heart rate.

Patients who do not have mechanical instability of the knee may tolerate walking without an increase in symptoms if they begin slowly and gradually increase their walking time to approximately 30 minutes 3 days a week. Each session should be preceded by a warm-up period consisting of ROM and strengthening exercises and followed by a cool-down period of stretching exercises. Because compliance with an exercise regimen is likely to decrease if pain increases, it is important to ascertain how much exercise is necessary to obtain the desired results and can be performed without producing significant pain.

Daily exercise which includes full, active ROM and periods of weight-bearing exercise appears to be necessary to maintain the integrity of articular cartilage. Even with preservation of ROM, loss of contraction of the periarticular muscles will lead to atrophy of the articular cartilage (Figures 1 and 2). When loading of the joint is contraindicated or immobilization is required, ROM exercises may help maintain some cartilage integrity.

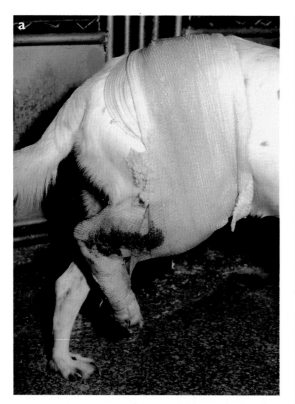

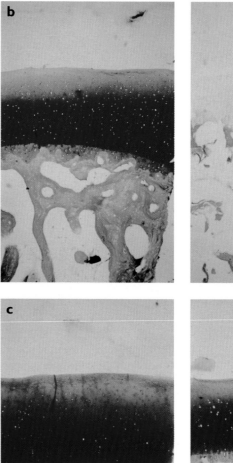

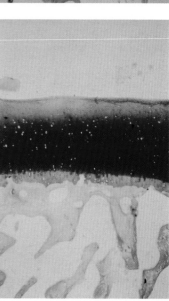

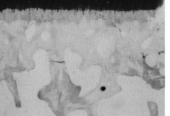

Figure 1 Loading is essential for maintenance of the integrity of a joint. (a) Immobilization of the hind limb of a normal dog in an orthopedic cast. (b) 3 months later marked atrophic changes have developed in both the articular cartilage and the bone (right hand panel). Note the loss of staining with safranin-O, reflecting the loss of cartilage proteoglycans. The surface of the articular cartilage is intact. (The pathology reflects cartilage atrophy, not OA.) Note also the marked disuse osteoporosis in the subchondral bone. For comparison, the histologic section on the left depicts the normal articular cartilage and subchondral bone in the contralateral (non-immobilized) knee. (c) After 12 weeks of immobilization, removal of the cast and ambulation *ad libitum* result in prompt and complete reversal of the changes of atrophy, and complete restitution of all of the associated structural, biochemical and metabolic changes in the cartilage

Many physicians fail to appreciate that a patient with OA is often able to tolerate load-bearing exercises and that an exercise program may decrease joint pain as much as treatment with a drug. Several studies have shown that a patient with hip or knee OA can participate safely in appropriate conditioning exercise programs to improve fitness and health without increasing joint pain or their requirement for analgesics or NSAIDs. Furthermore, in such studies, subject retention has been good and exercise behaviors have been maintained long after completion of the study protocol.

Exercise for health maintenance need not be as intensive as was previously believed. An effective exercise program can be designed even for those with significant joint disease.

Aerobic exercise

Regular physical activity is important for patients with knee OA. A subject with OA is less active and tends to be less fit with respect to both musculoskeletal and cardiovascular status than normal age- and sex-matched control subjects. The health benefits of aerobic exercise include increased aerobic capacity, muscle strength and exercise endurance, less exertion at a given work load, and weight loss.

In a randomized, controlled trial of aerobic exercise in 80 patients with symptomatic hip or knee OA, patients were randomized into three treatment groups for a 12-week program of aerobic walking, aerobic pool exercises, or non-aerobic ROM exercises. Both aerobic exercise groups showed significant improvement in aerobic capacity in comparison with the control group, and all three groups showed similar improvement with regard to joint pain and tenderness. Notably, no increase in the use of pain medication occurred in any of the three groups throughout the study period.

Another randomized, controlled trial of fitness walking in patients with knee OA employed an 8-week walking program which included flexibility and strengthening exercises as a warm-up and gradual progression of walking under supervision for 5 to 30 minutes 3 times per week. The control group received only a weekly telephone call. The walking group showed significant improvement with respect to walking distance, self-reported physical activity, and joint pain in comparison with the controls.

Aerobic exercises that may be recommended include walking, biking, swimming, aerobic dance, and aerobic pool exercises. Swimming and pool exercises cause less joint stress than the other forms of aerobic exercise. Each aerobic session should be preceded by a warm-up period consisting of ROM exercises and should be followed by a cool-down period of stretching. If walking or jogging results in an increase in symptoms, the patient should reduce the intensity of the activity or change to another form of aerobic exercise. Proper footwear is important and exercise on soft surfaces should be encouraged. To increase aerobic capacity, patients need to

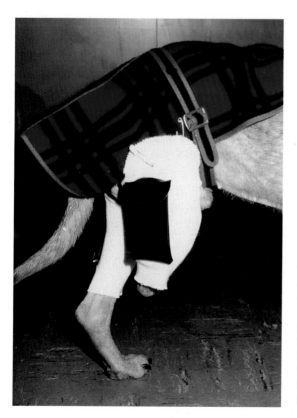

Figure 2 The changes induced by immobilization are due to a reduction in loading of the knee by contraction of the periarticular muscles (hamstrings, quadriceps), which normally occurs during the stance phase of gait. In the photograph, an activity displacement monitor is housed in the black pouch attached to the hind limb. The hip and knee are intact and the range of motion of those joints is essentially normal. However, because this dog has undergone an amputation of the paw, there is no stance phase of gait, and contraction of the periarticular muscles is markedly reduced. Changes in articular cartilage and bone in the ipsilateral knee after loss of the paw are essentially identical to those seen after immobilization, emphasizing the importance of the periarticular muscles in maintaining the integrity of joint tissues

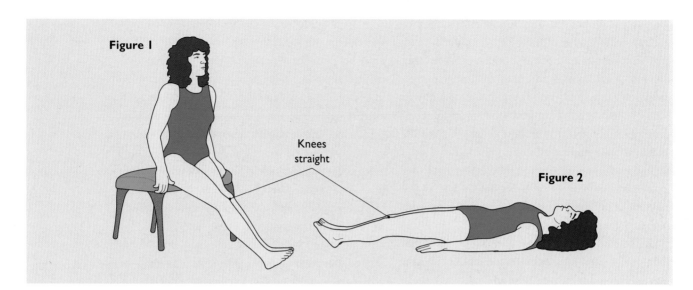

Figure 1

Knees straight

Figure 2

Table 1 Quadriceps strengthening exercise

1 Sit on a firm surface **(Figure 1)** or lie flat in bed **(Figure 2)**

2 Perform this exercise in either of the following positions:

   (a) Sit in a chair **(Figure 1)** with your legs straight, heels on the floor or on a footstool. Squeeze your thigh muscles, pushing your knees downward toward the floor

   (b) Lie in bed **(Figure 2)** with your legs straight and squeeze your thigh muscles, pushing the back of your knees into the bed

3 Hold this position for a full 5 seconds. Use a clock or watch with a second hand, or count: one-one thousand, two-one thousand, three-one thousand, four-one thousand, five-one thousand

4 Relax the muscles

5 Begin your strengthening program with 10 repetitions, holding each contraction for a full 5 seconds. Perform this exercise seven times daily and increase the number of repetitions you perform with each set by three to five daily during the first week

6 By the end of the week you should be able to perform 15 repetitions per set. This is the maximum number of repetitions you should perform in a set. (Total per day = 15 repetitions per set x 7 sets = 105)

7 If your arthritis is causing knee pain, apply heat to your knees for 15–20 minutes prior to performing your exercises

   Caution: In most patients, these knee exercises will not cause joint pain or increase the pain from your arthritis. If, however, you have significant pain lasting more than 20 minutes after you perform these exercises, decrease the number of repetitions by five per set. Maintain this number of repetitions until your knee discomfort subsides. Then, each day thereafter, increase the number of repetitions by three per set until you reach a maximum of 15 per set

From Rheumatology Division, Indiana University School of Medicine, 1993

Table 2 Quadriceps strengthening exercise concentrating on the vastus medialis oblique muscle

1 Sit on a firm surface **(Figure 1)** or lie flat in bed **(Figure 2)**

2 Cross your ankles with right leg above and left leg below. Legs should be stretched out straight

3 With your heels on the floor or on the bed, push down with right leg, push up with left leg, squeezing your ankles together. (Pretend that you're crushing a walnut between your ankles.) There should be little actual movement except for the muscle tightening

4 Hold this position for a full 5 seconds. Use a clock or watch with a second hand, or count: one-one thousand, two-one thousand, three-one thousand, four-one thousand, five-one thousand

5 Relax the muscles

6 Reverse the position of the legs so that the leg that was on top is now on the bottom

7 Repeat steps 1, 2 and 3

8 Begin your strengthening program with 10 repetitions, holding each contraction for a full 5 seconds. Perform this exercise seven times daily and increase the number of repetitions you perform with each set by three to five daily during the first week

9 By the end of the week you should be able to perform 15 repetitions per set. This is the maximum number of repetitions you should perform in a set. (Total per day = 15 repetitions per set x 7 sets = 105)

   Caution: In most patients, these knee exercises will not cause joint pain or increase the pain from your arthritis. If, however, you have significant pain lasting more than 20 minutes after you perform these exercises, decrease the number of repetitions by five per set. Maintain this number of repetitions until your knee discomfort subsides. Then, each day thereafter, increase the number of repetitions by three per set until you reach a maximum of 15 per set

From Rheumatology Division, Indiana University School of Medicine, 1993

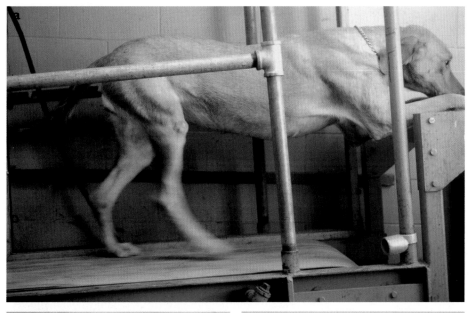

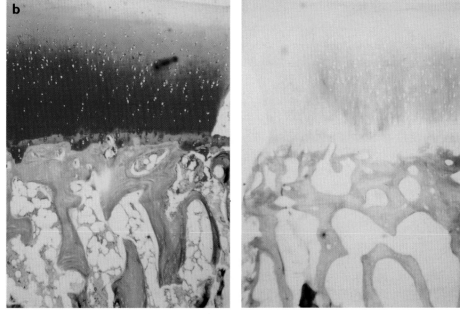

Figure 3 Overloading the extremity before the joint tissues have recovered from the effects of immobilization may result in irreversible joint damage. (a) Depicts a dog which underwent a 3-month period of immobilization, as in Figure 1. However, upon removal of the cast, the dog was placed on a treadmill exercise program, rather than being permitted to ambulate *ad libitum*. The level of activity was insufficient to produce damage to the normal canine joint. However, the loading imposed on the atrophic extremity resulted in permanent damage to the cartilage. (b) Proteoglycan synthesis increased several-fold upon remobilization but the newly synthesized cartilage matrix molecules were not effectively deposited and, because of permanent disruption of the collagen network of the cartilage, diffused into the joint space. The articular cartilage remained deficient in proteoglycans and, therefore, softer than normal after remobilization of the limb. The left hand panel depicts normal cartilage and subchondral bone from the contralateral (non-immobilized) knee

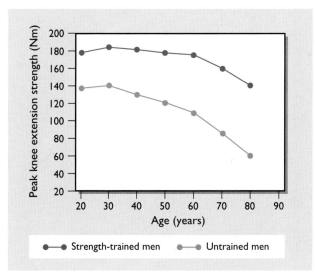

Figure 4 Changes in peak knee extensor strength in untrained and trained men at various ages. Even the elderly will show benefits of training. Reproduced with permission from Wilmore JH, Costill DL. Changes in strength with aging. In *Physiology of Sport and Exercise,* 2nd edn. Champaign: Human Kinetics, 1999:557

sustain a heart rate which is 60–80% of their target heart rate for 20 to 30 minutes 3 to 4 times weekly. Because maximum joint loading of the hip and knee occurs during stair climbing and descent, even though it is an excellent aerobic exercise, stair climbing may be inadvisable for a patient with OA affecting these joints.

Range of motion and strengthening exercises

Although aerobic exercise can increase aerobic power and reduce fatigue, it does not appear to improve muscle strength or functional capacity. Stretching or ROM exercises for a patient with OA seem to be helpful symptomatically, but controlled clinical trials have not been performed to document their value.

In the presence of knee OA, knee extensor strength may be diminished by as much as 60%. Exercise programs aimed at strengthening knee extension can result in significant gains in strength, reduction of joint pain and improvement in gait.

For strengthening, isometric exercises are recommended initially, because they employ less joint motion and are less likely to aggravate symptoms. Isometric quadriceps exercises, followed by progressive resistance exercises (which are superior to isometrics for maintaining or increasing function), will reduce joint pain and increase function in patients with knee OA. The intensity of the program should be increased gradually (Figure 3). Tables 1 and 2 contain instructions for isometric quadriceps exercises for patients with knee OA. The exercise which focuses on the vastus medialis obliquus muscle may be particularly helpful for a patient with lateral subluxation of the patella.

An exercise program aimed at strengthening knee extension should include training to increase contraction velocity and endurance as well as isometric and isotonic strength. Improvement in endurance and speed will result in much greater functional improvement than improvement in strength alone. A program of resistive strengthening of the hip, knee and ankle, coupled with postural control exercises, can result in significant improvement in strength and gait in older subjects with OA (Figures 4 and 5). The benefits of quadriceps strengthening exercise and aerobic exercise for patients with knee OA were confirmed recently in the Fitness Arthritis and Seniors Trial (FAST), in which patients with mild disability due to knee OA were randomized to either an aerobic exercise group, a resistance (muscle strengthening) exercise group, or an education/attention control group. Both exercise groups exhibited modest but significant improvement compared to the controls which, notably, was sustained over an 18 month period of observation.

Figure 5 Magnetic resonance imaging of the mid-thigh region of a subject before (a) and after (b) training. The subject was from a group of men, 85–92 years of age, who underwent training of the knee extensor and flexor muscles three times a week for 12 weeks. Reproduced with permission of John Wiley and Sons Inc., from Harridge SDR, Kryger A, Stensgaard A. Knee extensor strength, activation, and size in very elderly people following strength training. *Muscle Nerve* 1999;22:831–9

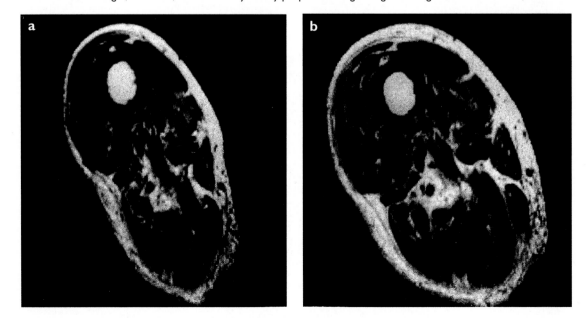

Exercise and joint protection

The periarticular muscles play a major role in attenuating shock to the joint. Attenuation of impact by neuromuscular mechanisms depends upon an adequate mass of conditioned muscle and the ability to generate force quickly for an eccentric contraction. As a consequence of pain or inactivity, muscle mass, contractile velocity, force production, endurance for repetitive motions, and motor skill all may be compromised in subjects with knee OA. To optimize a patient's neuromuscular capacity in order to protect the joint from sudden impact loading, exercises to improve concentric and eccentric strength and endurance at functional speeds and motor skill learning should be prescribed.

Because muscles are important shock absorbers and help stabilize the joint, periarticular muscle weakness may result in progression of structural damage to the joint in OA. In addition to the decrease in joint pain that exercise regimens which strengthen lower extremity muscles may achieve, they may also slow the progression of joint damage in patients with knee OA. Insufficient loading of a joint leads to atrophy of both the articular cartilage and subchondral bone. Control of loading is especially important for the joint with a weakened capsule, instability or muscle weakness severe enough to allow distortion of weight-bearing forces.

With respect to joint protection, the objectives of an exercise program are to reduce stress on the involved joint, improve shock attenuation during exercise and activities of daily living, and improve active joint motion and alignment. To control joint loading while preserving function, appropriate shoes, compliant walking surfaces (cinders, wood) and use of a cane, walker or crutches can all be helpful. In hip OA, use of a cane in the contralateral hand will reduce joint reaction forces by as much as 50%. Although such measurements have not been made in patients with knee OA, results should be similar. Furthermore, unloading the knee joint by use of a cane is often associated with a decrease in joint pain.

It has been shown that a simple exercise program can improve quadriceps strength, voluntary activation of the quadriceps muscle, proprioception, speed in performance of relevant function tests and scores on an algofunctional index in patients with knee OA, relative to controls who did

Table 3 Joint protection for patients with knee osteoarthritis

Recent studies show that protecting your arthritic knee from joint stress will decrease joint pain and protect your cartilage. Research has shown that ordinary walking transmits 3.5 times body weight across your knee cartilage; doing a squat puts a stress as high as 9 times body weight across your knee cartilage.

It is important that you protect your knees even if you are not experiencing joint pain. Sometimes, only simple adjustments are needed to improve your level of comfort and protect your joints. These are a few suggestions to help you protect your knees.

1   Wear properly fitted shoes with well-cushioned soles, such as Reeboks or Rockports. Sometimes special inserts are needed to readjust alignment and reduce stress on the knee. Your rheumatologist or physical therapist can help you decide what you need regarding footwear

2   Sit, rather than stand, for activities lasting longer than 10 minutes. When working at a counter for a lengthy period of time, sit on a high stool rather than stand. If you must stand, take at least a 5-minute break every hour

3   When arranging your work space, keep items that you use frequently where you can reach them easily without squatting or kneeling

4   A long-handled reacher can be used to pick up objects from the floor. This item can be obtained from the Occupational Therapy Department, a drug store that carries convalescent aids, or the Sears Home Health Catalog

5   Park your car close to your destination

6   Activities that jar your knees may further damage your cartilage. Swimming and walking will place much less stress on your knees than tennis, jogging or racquetball

7   Use ramps or elevators. If you must use stairs, take them one at a time, stopping occasionally to rest

8   Patients with knee arthritis should avoid:

   (a) Low chairs. Sit on a high, firm chair or use a pillow for elevation. Blocks can also be anchored under chair legs. This will put less stress on your knees and requires less energy when you stand up

   (b) Low beds. Blocks can be anchored under bed legs to increase the height of the bed

   (c) Low toilet seats. Elevated toilet seats, which will make getting up much easier, can be obtained from medical supply companies

   (d) Bathtubs. A shower with shower chair, if necessary, is a much better alternative

   (e) Kneeling, squatting or sitting cross-legged on the floor. All of these will put undue stress on your knee cartilage

From Rheumatology Division, Indiana University School of Medicine, 1993

Table 4   Application of heat to joint

The objective of applying heat to your arthritic joint is to reduce muscle spasm and joint pain. This may permit you to perform your joint exercises more effectively. You may find moist heat more effective than dry heat, although either can be used. Consider what is most convenient for you. You may use a shower or bath once a day, and use a heating pad for the other heat applications

Observe the following rules for safe and effective application of heat to your joints:

1   Apply heat to the affected area for no more than 15–20 minutes at a time

2   Avoid lying on a heating pad, since your body weight will decrease the circulation to that area and increase the risk of a burn

3   Before using a heating pad, wash off any liniment on the skin, since this could cause a burn

4   Use the heating pad only on low or medium temperature settings (not on high)

5   Do not apply heat to any region in which you have an artificial joint implanted

not participate in the program. Furthermore, the gains may persist for months after termination of the program.

In patients who had knee OA with varus deformity due to medial tibiofemoral compartment disease, treatment with an NSAID can result in a reduction in the severity of joint pain and increase in walking speed. However, these benefits may be accompanied by an increase in the adductor moment at the knee and greater loading of the damaged medial tibiofemoral compartment, in comparison with values obtained after an NSAID wash-out, when the patient is experiencing more pain. This increase in loading and increased stress on the supporting structures of the lateral aspect of the knee could, in the long run, outweigh the advantage of the increase in speed. Table 3 contains some general principles of joint protection for patients with knee OA.

Weight loss

The chapter on epidemiology emphasizes the importance of obesity as a risk factor for knee OA. Data also indicate that weight reduction in patients who are obese may result in a reduction in joint pain and improvement in function of weight-

bearing joints. Even a small amount of weight loss may be beneficial in patients with knee OA.

Thermal modalities

Applications of heat, cold or both have been widely employed for short-term pain relief in many musculoskeletal conditions, including OA. However, no controlled clinical trials of the application of superficial heat or cold to OA joints have been reported.

Heat

Most modalities for the application of superficial heat can elevate the temperature of the soft tissues 3°C at a depth of 1 cm beneath the surface. Thus, superficial heat applications do not penetrate deeper joints, such as the hip or knee; indeed, by diverting blood flow to more superficial tissues it may lower the intra-articular temperature slightly. However, a heat mitten for 30 minutes (i.e. longer than the usual duration of heat application for therapeutic purposes) may increase the temperature of the superficial small joints of the hand by 8°C.

Moist heat produces greater elevation of the subcutaneous temperature than dry heat and is often preferable for the relief of joint pain. With application of either dry or moist heat, care must be taken to avoid burning, particularly over bony prominences. Table 4 provides some practical instructions and precautions for a patient using application of heat to joints at home.

A patient with painful Heberden's nodes may find that dipping the hand into a paraffin bath is soothing and analgesic. Comparable results, however, may be obtained simply by immersing the hand in warm tap water. Hubbard tank hydrotherapy provides a generalized form of heat that permits simultaneous treatment of multiple painful joints and muscles. The buoyancy of the water is particularly useful in assuring that minimal stress will be applied to the joint during ROM exercises.

Deep heat is also useful and, in contrast to superficial heat, can affect the viscoelastic properties of collagen. Since tension is applied to the tissues as they are stretched, an increase in 'creep' (the plastic stretch of ligaments under tension) occurs. Application of deep heat prior to stretching

Figure 6 Medial taping of the patella may relieve pain in patients with patellofemoral osteoarthritis. Figure kindly provided by J. Cushnaghan, MSc, MCSP

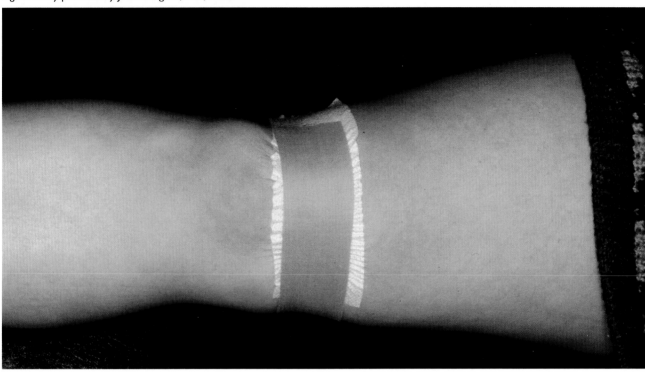

Figure 7 Lateral heel and sole wedge for treatment of knee pain in patients with medial tibiofemoral compartment osteoarthritis. Reproduced with permission of publisher, from Keating EM, Faris PM, Ritter MA, Kane J. Use of lateral heel and sole wedges in the treatment of medial osteoarthritis of the knee. *Orthop Rev* 1993;22:921–4 © 2000 Quadrant Healthcom Inc.

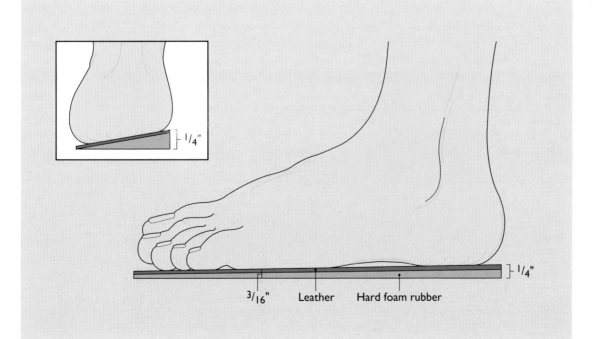

exercises will enhance the efficacy of the exercises. Ultrasound penetrates more deeply than either shortwave or microwave diathermy and, among these three forms of deep heat, it alone can raise the intra-articular temperature of the hip. Joint pain in a patient with OA of the hip or knee can be significantly reduced by either ultrasound or short-wave diathermy. Deep heat is contraindicated in a patient with a local malignancy or bleeding diathesis and after laminectomy. The risk of thermal injury with the use of any of the above heat modalities is increased if the circulation is poor, the patient is sedated, or sensation impaired.

Cold

Cold is often recommended to relieve muscle aching after strenuous exercise. It may be delivered by ice packs, ice massage or local spray. Superficial cooling can decrease muscle spasm and increase the pain threshold. Vapo-coolant sprays may be very effective over areas of painful muscle trigger points. Cold applications should not be used, however, in patients with Raynaud's phenomenon, cold hypersensitivity, cryoglobulinemia, or paroxysmal cold hemoglobinuria.

Patellar taping

OA of the patellofemoral compartment can cause severe pain, especially with kneeling, squatting or climbing stairs. Cushnaghan and colleagues reported a controlled clinical trial of knee taping to realign the patella in 14 subjects with patello-

femoral OA. Evidence of tibiofemoral joint OA was also present in all cases, but in the majority X-ray changes of OA were more severe in the patello-femoral compartment than in the tibiofemoral compartment. The results showed a significant reduction in pain for medial taping in comparison with taping in the lateral or neutral position. Furthermore, patient preference favored medial taping over the other positions. The decrease in pain appeared to be clinically, as well as statistically, significant.

The taping procedure is simple. Patients can learn to apply their own tape after minimal instruction (Figure 6). The treatment is inexpensive and can be controlled by the patient. The prompt relief of symptoms which may be achieved by the taping may be maintained by concurrent isometric exercises to strengthen the vastus medialis obliquus component of the quadriceps muscle, facilitating realignment of the patella on a long-term basis.

Wedged insoles

By reducing excessive loading on the medial compartment of the knee and strain on the lateral collateral ligament, wedged insoles may be useful in the conservative treatment of OA of the medial tibiofemoral compartment (Figure 7). In a comparative study of 107 patients with early radiographic changes of OA, 67 were treated with both the wedged insole and indomethacin, 60 mg/d, while 40 were treated with indomethacin alone. The insole group showed significantly greater improvement.

Table 5 Scores for pain and walking ability with use of a wedged insole in relation to radiographic severity of osteoarthritis

Radiographic stage of osteoarthritis	Number of patients	Pain score		Walking ability score	
		Before use	After use	Before use	After use
I	30	15.7 ± 9.7	10.7 ± 9.7	14.7 ± 5.9	3.0 ± 4.5
II	37	15.8 ± 9.3	10.4 ± 8.7	13.1 ± 4.7	4.6 ± 3.6
III	20	14.8 ± 5.3	7.0 ± 8.3	12.8 ± 3.8	3.0 ± 4.1
IV	15	11.0 ± 5.5	4.9 ± 10.1	11.0 ± 4.5	0.3 ± 3.4

Values represent means ± SD of pain scores and walking ability scores. The matched-pair t-test was used to test the significance of changes in scores. Student's t-test or the Fisher-Behrens test was used to test significance of the scores among the four stages of radiographic severity. Statistically significant differences in the walking ability score were noted between Stage II and Stage IV. Modified from Sasaki T, Yasuda K. Clinical evaluation of the treatment of osteoarthritic knees using a newly designed wedged insole. *Clin Orthop Rel Res* 1987;221:181–7

The insole was significantly more effective for patients with mild OA than for those with more advanced disease (Table 5). The data suggest that the wedged insole represents an effective, conservative treatment for early, medial compartment knee OA.

In an uncontrolled study, Keating and colleagues found lateral heel and sole wedges to be effective even in some patients with complete loss of medial compartment joint space on their knee X-ray. Fifty per cent of the 85 patients evaluated (121 knees) showed an improvement in pain score of a magnitude corresponding to a good result from total knee arthroplasty. As noted in the study cited above, patients with milder OA received greater pain relief than those with more severe disease. However, even marked loss of joint space did not preclude a good result. A polypropylene mesh shoe-type insole is practical, inexpensive, washable and will last approximately 2 years, i.e. twice as long as a leather insole.

Patient education

Patient education programs offer benefits beyond those of NSAIDs in the symptomatic treatment of patients with OA. A meta-analysis found that patient education interventions resulted in an additional benefit 20–30% as large as the effect of NSAID treatment alone. Mazzuca *et al.*, found that self-care education for inner-city patients with knee OA (i.e. a group with relatively poor social support) resulted in preservation of function and control of knee pain. For effective management of many patients with OA, encouragement, reassurance, advice about exercise and recommendation of measures to unload the arthritic joint (e.g. a cane, proper footwear) may be all that is required.

Bibliography

Blair SN, Kohl HW, Gordon NF, Paffenbarger RS Jr. How much physical activity is good for health? *Ann Rev Public Health* 1992;13:99–126

Cushnaghan J, McCarthy C, Dieppe P. Taping the patella medially: a new treatment for osteoarthritis of the knee joint? *Br Med J* 1994;308:753

Ettinger WH Jr, Burns R, Messier SP, et al. A randomized trial comparing aerobic exercise and resistance exercise with a health education program in older adults with knee osteoarthritis. The Fitness Arthritis and Senior Trial (FAST). *JAMA* 1997;227:25–31

Felson DT, Anderson JJ, Naimark A, et al. Obesity and knee osteoarthritis. The Framingham Study. *Ann Intern Med* 1998;109:18–24

Fisher NM, Pendergast DR, Gresham GE, Calkins E. Muscle rehabilitation: its effect on muscular and functional performance of patients with knee osteoarthritis. *Arch Phys Med Rehabil* 1991;72:367–74

Hollander JL, Horvath SM. Changes in joint temperature produced by diseases and by physical therapy. *Arch Phys Med Rehabil* 1949;30:437–40

Jeusevar DS, Riley PO, Hodge WA, Krebs DE. Knee kinematics and kinetics during locomotor activities of daily living in subjects with knee arthroplasty and in healthy controls. *Phys Ther* 1993;73:229–42

Kovar PA, Allegrante JP, Mackenzie CR, et al. Supervised fitness walking in patients with osteoarthritis of the knee: a randomized, controlled trial. *Ann Intern Med* 1992;116:529–34

Mazzuca SA, Brandt KD, Katz BP, et al. Effects of self-care education on the health status of inner-city patients with osteoarthritis of the knee. *Arthritis Rheum* 1997;40:1466–74

Minor M. Exercise in the management of osteoarthritis of the knee and hip. *Arthritis Care Res* 1994;7:198–204

Palmoski MJ, Colyer RA, Brandt KD. Joint motion in the absence of normal loading does not maintain normal articular cartilage. *Arthritis Rheum* 1980;23:325–34

Radin EL, Yang KH, Riegger C, et al. Relationship between lower limb dynamics and knee joint pain. *J Orthoped Res* 1991;9:398–405

Schnitzer TJ, Popovich JM, Andersson GBJ, Andriacchi TP. Effect of piroxicam on gait in patients with osteoarthritis of the knee. *Arthritis Rheum* 1993;36:1207–13

Superio-Cabuslay E, Ward MM, Korig KR. Patient education interventions in osteoarthritis and rheumatoid arthritis: a meta-analytic comparison with nonsteroidal antiinflammatory drug treatment. *Arthritis Care Res* 1996;9:292–301

Yasuda K, Sasaki T. The mechanics of treatment of the osteoarthritic knee with a wedged insole. *Clin Orthop* 1987; 215:162–72

CHAPTER ELEVEN

Systemic pharmacologic therapy

1. Acetaminophen and NSAIDs

Acetaminophen

The efficacy of acetaminophen (ACET) in palliation of osteoarthritis pain

The evidence indicates that a simple analgesic may be as effective as an NSAID in symptomatic treatment of many patients with osteoarthritis. In a study of patients with chronic knee pain and moderately severe radiographic changes of OA treated for 4 weeks with either an anti-inflammatory dose or analgesic dose of ibuprofen (2400 mg/d, 1200 mg/d, respectively), or with ACET (4000 mg/d), we found no superiority of either the anti-inflammatory dose or the lower dose of ibuprofen, in comparison with ACET (Table 1). Even the presence of clinical features of synovitis (e.g. joint swelling, synovial effusion, synovial tenderness) did not predict a better response to the anti-inflammatory regimen than to ACET. Similarly, no significant difference was found between the NSAID flurbiprofen, and the analgesic, nefopam, in patients with symptomatic knee OA. Furthermore, ibuprofen in a daily dose of only 1200 mg (which, as noted above, provides only a weak anti-inflammatory effect) was as effective as several other NSAIDs, including the very potent anti-inflammatory drug phenylbutazone (Table 2), in relieving joint pain in patients with OA, even when the others were given in anti-inflammatory doses.

What about the severity of joint pain as a determinant of the response to an NSAID versus an analgesic? In a retrospective study of patients with knee OA who were treated with either an anti-inflammatory dose of ibuprofen, an analgesic dose of ibuprofen or acetaminophen, neither the severity of general arthritis pain, rest pain or walking pain at baseline predicted a better clinical response to the anti-inflammatory regimen than to the analgesic regimens

Studies of NSAID withdrawal further justify the consideration of alternatives to chronic NSAID therapy in the elderly. For example: nearly 50% of

Table 1 Clinical outcomes in patients with knee joint tenderness or swelling at baseline exam

	Acetaminophen 4000 mg/d n=43	Ibuprofen 1200 mg/d n=39	2400 mg/d n=42	p value
HAQ disability*	0.0 ± 0.3	0.1 ± 0.4	0.1 ± 0.5	0.94
HAQ pain*	0.5 ± 0.7	0.3 ± 0.9	0.3 ± 1.0	0.54
Rest pain*	0.1 ± 0.6	0.4 ± 0.8	0.4 ± 1.1	0.16
Walk pain*	0.1 ± 0.7	0.3 ± 0.9	0.5 ± 1.0	0.20
50-ft walk time*	0.5 ± 1.6	0.5 ± 4.2	0.6 ± 3.7	0.97
% improved**	33%	48%	33%	0.13

*Improvement in score with treatment, relative to the baseline value, mean ± standard deviation. Analyzed using ANOVA. HAQ, Health Assessment Questionnaire. **Physician's Global Assessment of change in the patient's arthritis was analyzed using a Chi-squared test. Modified from Bradley JD, Brandt KD, Katz BP, et al. Treatment of knee osteoarthritis: relationship of clinical features of joint inflammation to the response to a nonsteroidal anti-inflammatory drug or pure analgesic. J Rheumatol 1992;19:1950–4

Table 2 Improvement, initial to end of week 4

	Ibuprofen 300 mg qid		Phenylbutazone 100 mg qid		χ^2 p
Overall disease state	26/76	(34.2%)	30/70	(42.9%)	NS
Exercise and related pain	47/77	(61.0%)	50/70	(71.4%)	NS
Performance of selected activities	47/72	(65.3%)	51/62	(82.3%)	NS
Physician's assessment	30/71	(42.3%)	30/63	(47.6%)	NS

An analgesic dose of ibuprofen (1200 mg/d) was as effective as the very potent anti-inflammatory drug phenylbutazone, 400 mg/d, in providing symptomatic relief for patients with knee OA. From Moxley TE, Royer GL, Hearron MS, *et al.* Ibuprofen versus buffered phenylbutazone in the treatment of osteoarthritis: double blind trial. *J Am Geriatr Soc* 1975;23:343–9

Table 3 NSAID withdrawal in the elderly

	Patients
Admitted on NSAID	91
NSAID withdrawn	78 (86%)
Alive and off NSAID	
at 4 weeks	45/67 (67%)
at 6 months	36/67 (54%)

From Black D, Tuppen J, Heller A. NSAID withdrawal in elderly patients. *J Am Geriatr Soc* 1991;39:A26

hospitalized geriatric patients who were regular NSAID users were withdrawn successfully and, upon review 6 months later, had not required further NSAID treatment (Table 3).

For the above reasons and, particularly, because of concern about side-effects of NSAIDs (see below), recent American College of Rheumatology guidelines for the management of hip OA and knee OA recommend ACET, in a dose of up to 4000 mg/d, as the initial drug for the symptomatic treatment of OA. This recommendation was reinforced with the publication of an update to the ACR guidelines in November 2000.

Side-effects of ACET

Hepatotoxicity

Side-effects of ACET are uncommon and generally mild. Although, in the case of overdose, ACET can cause hepatotoxicity and even acute hepatic necrosis with fulminant hepatic failure, this has generally been seen with daily doses exceeding 10 g, i.e. 2.5 times the maximum recommended therapeutic

Figure 1 Pathways for metabolism of acetaminophen. While most of the drug is conjugated with glucuronide or sulfate in the liver, some is metabolized through the cytochrome p450 enzyme system, producing the highly reactive metabolite, NAPQI. In the presence of adequate stores of glutathione, a harmless metabolite is produced. However, if NAPQI concentrations are increased or a relative deficiency of glutathione exists (e.g. as a result of alcoholism), NAPQI interacts with intracellular macromolecules, resulting in cell damage and death. Glucuronidation may be impaired by glycogen depletion (e.g. in starvation), diverting more metabolism along the potentially toxic p450 pathway

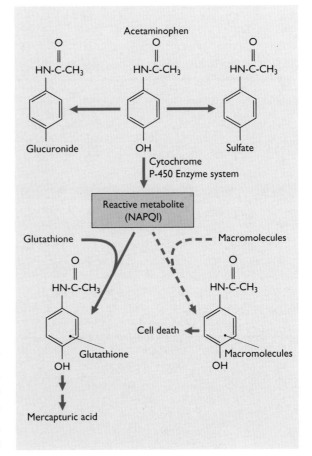

dose for adults. Regular consumption of alcohol lowers the threshold for ACET-induced liver damage by inducing the enzymes that catalyze metabolism of the drug, leading to an increase in concentration of the toxic metabolite *N*-acetyl-p-benzo-quinone-imine (NAPQI, Figure 1). The syndrome is characterized by a striking elevation of the serum asparate aminotransferase (AST) level and a fatality rate of approximately 20%. It is prudent to discourage regular use of any analgesic in patients who consume alcohol regularly and to encourage use of the lowest possible dose by those who use analgesics regularly.

Renal disease

Few reports exist of ACET-induced renal disease, presumably because of the absence of peripheral inhibition of prostaglandin synthesis. Acute ACET nephrotoxicity has been documented only with overdoses, when it is most often secondary to acute hepatic failure.

A National Kidney Foundation position paper states: 'ACET remains the non-narcotic analgesic of choice for episodic use in patients with underlying renal disease' but 'habitual consumption of ACET should be discouraged [and when] indicated medically, long-term use of this drug should be supervised by a physician'.

Nonsteroidal anti-inflammatory drugs (NSAIDs)

NSAIDs are analgesic, anti-inflammatory and antipyretic drugs and have as their predominant mechanism of action the inhibition of the enzyme cyclo-oxygenase, which plays a critical role in prostaglandin biosynthesis. The adverse effects of this class of drugs on, for example, the gastro-intestinal tract, kidney and platelets are also due to prostaglandin inhibition. It is now recognized that two isoforms of cyclo-oxygenase exist and that the adverse effects of NSAIDs are due predominantly (although not exclusively) to inhibition of the synthesis of one isoform while the beneficial effects are due to inhibition of synthesis of the other isoform.

Short-term efficacy of NSAIDs in osteoarthritis

There is ample evidence that NSAIDs are superior to placebo for symptomatic treatment of osteo-arthritis. However, their effect is only modest and

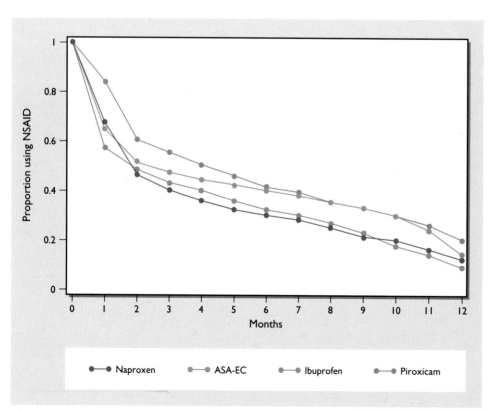

Figure 2 Among patients with osteoarthritis who were started on an NSAID, only about 15%, on average, were still on the same NSAID 12 months later. ASA-EC, enteric-coated aspirin. Scholes D, Stergachis A, Penna PM, *et al.* Nonsteroidal antiinflammatory drug discontinuation in patients with osteoarthritis. *J Rheumatol* 1995;22:708–12

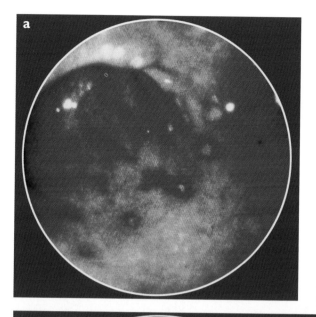

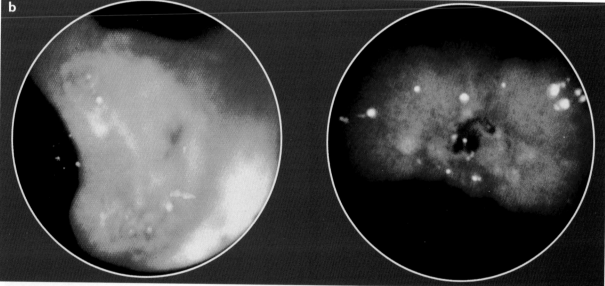

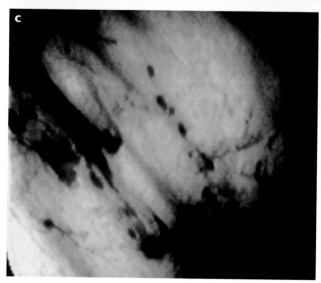

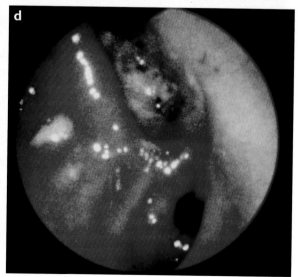

Figure 3 (a) Multiple gastric erosions, seen endoscopically. These lesions, which develop commonly with the use of nonselective NSAIDs, are superficial and small (generally ≤3 mm in diameter). They are often asymptomatic and do not appear to bear any relationship to serious gastric adverse events, such as hemorrhage, perforation and obstruction. From the Slide Collection of the American College of Gastroenterology. (b) Gastric ulcer, with a blood vessel apparent in the fibrinous base of the lesion. In contrast to erosions, gastric (and duodenal) ulcers in NSAID users are larger (≥5 mm), penetrate the muscularis mucosa, and may be associated with clinically important adverse events, such as hemorrhage, perforation and obstruction. From the Slide Collection of the American College of Gastroenterology. (c) Mucosal hemorrhages in the stomach of another patient taking a nonselective NSAID. Some of the individual lesions are petechial, while others are considerably larger. Photograph kindly provided by David Bjorkman, MD. (d) Large gastric ulcer seen endoscopically in another patient taking a nonselective NSAID. Note the grey fibrinous base of the ulcer and bleeding immediately beneath the surface. Photograph kindly provided by David Bjorkman, MD

Figure 4 Number of deaths associated with NSAID-induced gastrointestinal damage compared to those from other causes in the United States population, 1997. A total of 16 500 patients with rheumatoid arthritis or OA died from gastrointestinal effects of NSAIDs. From Singh G, Triadafilopoulos G. Epidemiology of NSAID induced gastrointestinal complications. *J Rheumatol* 1999;26 (Suppl 56):18–24

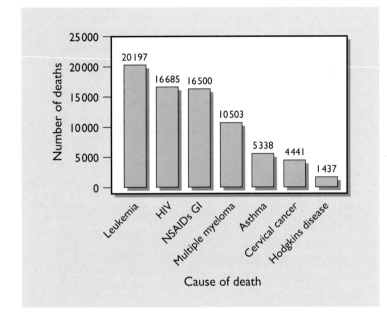

Figure 5 Effects of aspirin treatment at 10 mg/d (*n* = 8), 81mg/d (*n* = 11), and 325 mg/d (*n* = 10) on endoscopic injury scores in the stomach, duodenum and rectum, expressed as change (± SEM) from the baseline value. Data obtained after 1.5 months and 3 months were averaged. For the rectum, *n* = 7 for each aspirin dose. No rectal biopsies were performed at 1.5 months. *$p \leq 0.05$ vs. baseline by the Wilcoxon signed-rank test. Reproduced with permission from Cryer B, Feldman M. Effects of very low dose daily, long-term aspirin therapy on gastric, duodenal, and rectal prostaglandin levels and on mucosal injury in healthy humans. *Gastroenterology* 1999;117:17–25

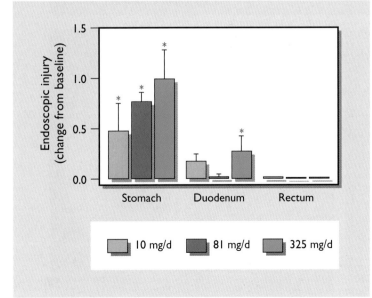

Table 4 Risk factors for upper gastrointestinal adverse events in patients taking NSAIDs

Increasing age
Comorbidity (poor or fair general health)
Oral glucocorticoids
History of peptic ulcer disease
History of upper gastrointestinal bleeding
Anticoagulation
Combination NSAID therapy
Increasing NSAID dose
Smoking (?)
Alcohol (?)

control of symptoms is rarely complete. Furthermore, for many patients they are not clearly superior to ACET and a substantial proportion of OA patients receiving chronic NSAID therapy may do as well with withdrawal of their NSAID and use of ACET only as needed. It is not surprising that only about 15% of patients with OA for whom an NSAID is prescribed are still using the same NSAID 12 months later (Figure 2).

Major adverse effects of non-selective NSAIDS

NSAID gastroenteropathy

Much of the current ambivalence of physicians with respect to NSAID administration in OA is related to concern about the adverse effects of these agents, especially those related to the gastrointestinal (GI) tract. Prospective controlled studies have shown a relative risk of about 1.5 for perforation or hemorrhage of an NSAID-related peptic ulcer; in case-control studies the relative risk has been 3 to 4 times higher (Figure 3). In particular, those at greatest risk for OA, i.e. the elderly, are also at greatest risk for gastrointestinal symptoms, ulceration, hemorrhage and death.

Among elderly individuals the annual rate of hospitalization for peptic ulcer disease (PUD) among current NSAID users is 16/1000 – four times greater than that for subjects not taking an NSAID. The risk increases with the dose; the annual hospitalization rate rises from 4/1000 for those who did not use NSAIDs to more than 40/1000 for those using the highest doses. The risk of serious gastrointestinal complications among patients with OA who take NSAIDs for one year has been found to be 7.3 per 1000. It was estimated that 16 500 NSAID-related deaths now occur annually, among patients with rheumatoid arthritis or OA, in the United States, a number similar to that of deaths from acquired immune deficiency syndrome (AIDS) and considerably greater than the death toll from multiple myeloma, asthma, cervical cancer or Hodgkin's disease (Figure 4). Among people aged 65 years and older, as many as 30% of all hospitalizations and deaths related to PUD can be attributed to NSAID use.

Not only serious and life-threatening adverse GI events, such as perforation, ulceration and upper GI hemorrhage, but nonspecific GI adverse events, such as dyspepsia, abdominal pain and diarrhea, are associated with NSAID use. The latter, even if not life-threatening, are important because they affect compliance with prescribed NSAID dosing and result in the use of additional therapies for treatment of the symptoms, thereby increasing the cost

Table 5 Prevalence of drug use among patients with upper gastrointestinal hemorrhage

	Number of patients (% ± 95% CI)
OTC aspirin	145 (35 ± 4.6)
OTC non-aspirin NSAID	36 (9 ± 2.7)
Prescription aspirin	27 (6 ± 2.4)
Prescription non-aspirin NSAID	56 (14 ± 3.3)
OTC aspirin and non-aspirin NSAID	20 (5 ± 2.1)
Any aspirin	170 (41 ± 4.8)
Any non-aspirin NSAID	90 (22 ± 2.2)
Any drug	229 (56 ± 4.8)

Some patients took more than one drug. Prescription and over-the-counter (OTC) drug use was unknown in 8 patients and 10 patients, respectively; CI, confidence interval. Reproduced with permission from Wilcox CM, Shalek KA, Cotsonis G. Striking prevalence of over-the-counter nonsteroidal antiinflammatory drug use in patients with upper gastrointestinal hemorrhage. *Arch Intern Med* 1999;154:42–6; copyrighted 1994, American Medical Association

Table 6 Effects of inhibition of prostaglandin synthesis in the presence of various antihypertensive drugs

Class of antihypertensive	Primary mode of action	Effect of blocking prostaglandin synthesis
Diuretic	↓ extracellular volume and total peripheral resistance	↓ loss of salt and water, exacerbated in presence of low plasma renin activity
Beta-adrenergic blocker	Inhibit secretion of renin→ ↓ in angiotensin and aldosterone	Inhibit renin release, may limit ability to reduce plasma renin activity
		Propranolol stimulates PGI_2 synthesis in patients with essential hypertension
ACE inhibitor	Inhibit formation of angiotensin II and aldosterone, inhibit inactivitation of bradykinin	Interfere with release of bradykinin (which is mediated through local prostaglandin release)
Vasodilator	Unclear – thought to act through prostaglandin mediated mechanisms	May interfere with prostaglandin-mediated mechanisms
Central alpha$_2$-agonist	↓ sympathetic output from the CNS →↓ in cardiac output and peripheral resistance	May ↑ total peripheral resistance
Peripheral alpha$_1$-adrenergic blocker	Inhibit vasoconstriction induced by endogenous catecholamines	Potential attenuation of vasodilatory effect
	Prazosin stimulates formation of PGI_2 and PGE_2 *in vitro*	
Angiotensin II blocker	Block peripheral vasoconstriction and renal salt-sparing action of angiotensin II	In studies in animals, action of losartan was unaffected by inhibition of prostaglandin synthesis
		In the same animal model, prostaglandin inhibition blocked angiotensin II-mediated ↑ in GFR

PG, prostaglandin; ACE, angiotensin-converting enzyme; CNS, central nervous system; GFR, glomerular filtration rate. Reproduced with permission from Ruoff GE. The impact of nonsteroidal anti-inflammatory drugs on hypertension: alternative analgesics for patients at risk. *Clin Ther* 1998;20:376–87 and Whelton A. Renal and related cardiovascular effects of conventional and Cox-2 specific NSAIDs and non-NSAID analgesics. *Am J Therapeutics* 2000;7:63–74

of managing the disease and, at times, producing additional side-effects.

Dyspepsia correlates poorly with the presence of endoscopically visualized lesions or clinical episodes of GI bleeding. Most patients who incur serious GI complications from NSAID use have not had prior GI symptoms. In addition to age and dose, risk factors associated with NSAID-induced peptic ulcer complications are shown in Table 4.

With respect to the risk associated with anti-coagulants, not only warfarin but aspirin – even in the low doses used for cardiovascular prophylaxis – may cause problems. Even 10 mg of aspirin/d may lead to GI complications. In normal volunteers, this dose significantly reduced gastric mucosal prosta-glandin levels to about 40% of the baseline value and induced gastric injury (Figure 5). A dose of 325 mg/day also resulted in duodenal injury. Although a 10 mg dose did not significantly reduce duodenal mucosal prostaglandin levels, 81 mg and 325 mg resulted in reductions to about 40% of the baseline value. Serum thromboxane (TBXA$_2$) levels were inhibited by 62%, 90% and 98%, respectively, with a daily dose of 10 mg, 81 mg and 325 mg of aspirin.

Histamine$_2$ (H$_2$) receptor antagonists reduce the incidence of endoscopically-diagnosed NSAID-induced duodenal ulcer. Omeprazole reduced the incidence of NSAID-induced gastric ulcer and miso-prostol, a prostaglandin E$_1$ analog, reduced the inci-dence of both. That this decrease in endoscopically recognizable ulcers may be accompanied by a decrease in the rate of GI perforation, hemorrhage, and death is suggested by the results of a 6-month, randomized, double-blind, placebo-controlled trial involving nearly 9000 patients with rheumatoid arthritis, in which misoprostol reduced the risk of serious upper GI complications of NSAID use by 40%. However, despite the very large number of sub-jects enrolled, the reduction in risk barely reached statistical significance ($p=0.049$).

Routine co-prescription of misoprostol with NSAIDs is controversial. Misoprostol is expensive and, as indicated above, its efficacy is by no means complete. Furthermore diarrhea is relatively common with misoprostol, and it often does not relieve NSAID-induced dyspepsia. Therefore the daily quality of life of patients taking misoprostol may be worse than that of those taking an NSAID

alone. Certainly, for that subgroup of OA patients at high risk for ulcer complications, in whom sympto-matic benefit from an NSAID is significantly greater than that from a nonacetylated salicylate or an analgesic, it is reasonable to prescribe misoprostol. However, many patients will not tolerate the recommended dose of 200 µg qid. A dose of 200 µg bid is better tolerated, but affords significantly less protection from gastric ulcers.

As an alternative to misoprostol an H$_2$-receptor antagonist, e.g. famotidine, or a proton pump inhibitor, e.g. omeprazole, may be used. Both have been shown by endoscopy to be effective in treating and preventing NSAID-induced ulcers, although the protective effect of neither has been assessed in large-scale clinical trials. However, in usual doses, H$_2$ blockers were not as effective as misoprostol in treatment of existing ulcers whereas omeprazole, 20 or 40 mg/d, was as effective as a 200 µg bid dose of misoprostol, better tolerated and associated with a lower relapse rate.

GI hemorrhage is associated not only with the prescription use of NSAIDs, but also with over-the-counter (OTC) use. In a recent study of 421 patients who were evaluated for upper GI hemorrhage, use of an OTC aspirin or nonaspirin NSAID during the week prior to admission was reported by 35% and 9%, respectively, while prescription use of a nonaspirin NSAID or aspirin was reported in much lower proportions – 14% and 6% respectively (Table 5). Given the high frequency with which these OTC agents are used, short-time NSAID use may be a major cause of ulcer-related hemorrhage.

In addition to their adverse effects on the gastric and duodenal mucosa, NSAIDs have been associated with deleterious effects on the small intestine, including inflammation associated with loss of blood and protein, stricture ulceration, perforation and diarrhea. NSAIDs also cause large bowel perforation and hemorrhage. Clinical mani-festations of the effects of NSAIDs on the small and large bowel, however, are much less frequent than upper GI tract problems.

Cardiovascular–renal effects of NSAIDS

Inhibition of prostaglandin biosynthesis by NSAIDs is also a well recognized cause of other common, and occasionally severe, side-effects, including

Table 7 Risk factors for NSAID-induced renal disease

Pre-existing renal disease
Diabetes mellitus
Hypertension
Congestive heart failure
Cirrhosis
Volume depletion (due e.g. to diuretics, hemorrhage, diarrhea, profuse sweating)

hypertension, congestive heart failure, hyperkalemia and renal insufficiency. Many antihypertensive drugs exert their therapeutic effect, in part, through prostaglandin-mediated mechanisms (Table 6). Although NSAIDs generally have little or no effect on blood pressure in normotensive individuals, they may increase blood pressure in hypertensive patients under treatment. While the increase may be only some 4–5 mmHg, it should be noted that an increase in diastolic blood pressure of as little as 5–6 mmHg over a few years may increase the risk of a cerebrovascular accident by 67% and of coronary artery disease by 15%, while a decline in elevated diastolic blood pressure may decrease the incidence of stroke and congestive heart failure by nearly 40% and 25%, respectively. Among elderly patients who were taking diuretics, concomitant use of an NSAID doubled the risk of hospitalization for congestive heart failure.

Figure 6 depicts the consequences of inhibition of prostaglandin levels in the kidney, such as sodium and water retention, hyperkalemia and renal failure. Patients at greatest risk for renal complications of NSAIDs include those with pre-existing renal disease, hypertension, congestive heart failure, cirrhosis, and volume depletion as may occur with the use of diuretics, hemorrhage, diarrhea, or profuse sweating (Table 7). Even a dose of NSAID so low that it has minimal anti-inflammatory effects may lead to renal insufficiency.

While acute effects on renal blood flow in NSAID users are much more common than chronic

Figure 6 Renal effects associated with NSAID-induced prostaglandin inhibition. Reproduced with permission from Aronoff GR. Therapeutic implications associated with renal studies of nabumetone. *J Rheumatol* 1992;19(suppl 36):25–31

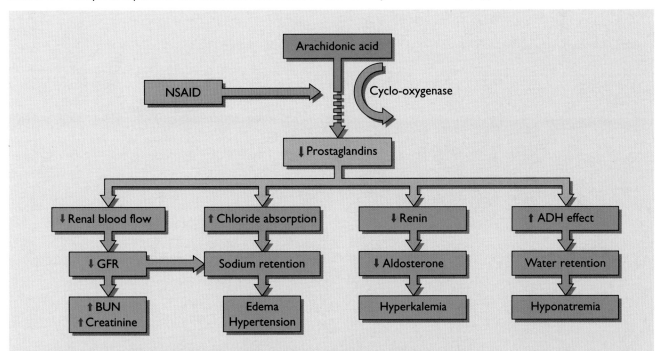

GFR = glomerular filtration rate;   BUN = blood urea nitrogen;   ADH = antidiuretic hormone

renal changes, NSAIDs can cause chronic renal disease. Indeed, they are much more likely to do so than ACET. The increased risk for chronic renal disease, which is largely confined to men over 65 years of age, results in an odds ratio of 16:1 for daily NSAID use.

Acute interstitial nephritis, with new onset proteinuria, usually in the nephrotic range, may occur at any time during NSAID therapy, although its prevalence is only 0.01–0.02%. Histologic examination shows minimal change in glomerulonephritis and interstitial nephritis. The problem usually remits within weeks after discontinuation of the NSAID, but resolution may take many months. Whelton has recently provided an excellent review of the renal effects of NSAIDs and analgesics.

Do NSAIDs alter the rate of cartilage breakdown in osteoarthritis?

A number of reports suggest that NSAIDs may slow the progression of cartilage breakdown in OA, thus serving as disease-modifying OA drugs (DMOADs). Such claims, however, have been based largely on *in vitro* effects of the drug on cytokine production, release or activity of cartilage matrix-degrading proteases, inhibition of the production of toxic oxygen metabolites, etc. There are no data from controlled clinical trials in humans to indicate that any NSAID favorably influences progression of joint breakdown in OA. Indeed, several NSAIDs inhibit proteoglycan (PG) synthesis by normal cartilage *in vitro* (Figure 7). Because PGs are essential for the elasticity and compressive stiffness of cartilage,

Figure 7 Effects of some NSAIDs on incorporation of ^{35}S into organ cultures of normal canine articular cartilage. Some NSAIDs inhibit glycosaminoclycans synthesis *in vitro*, others have essentially no effect, while yet others stimulate synthesis *in vitro*. The concentrations of drugs shown in the figure approximate those which are achievable in serum or synovial fluid of patients treated with the respective NSAID. From Brandt KD, Palmoski MJ. Effects of salicylates and other nonsteroidal anti-inflammatory drugs on articular cartilage. *Am J Med* 1984;77:65–9

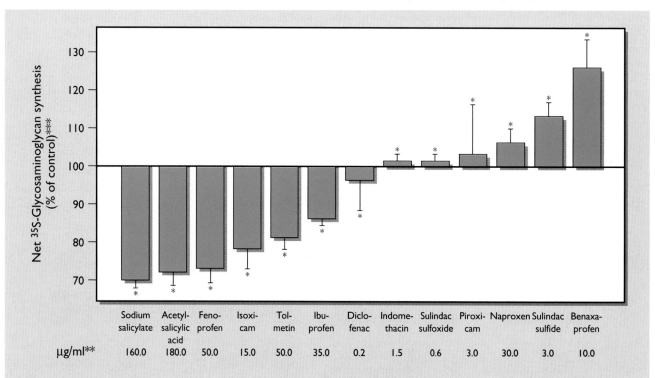

* *p* < 0.01 compared to control.
** Corresponds to plasma concentration achieved in humans with oral administration of the drug.
*** Non-dialyzable ^{35}SO$_4$ cpm in medium and pronase digest/10 mg wet weight of cartilage. Mean ± 1 SE.

suppression of their synthesis *in vivo* could have adverse consequences. The augmented *in vitro* synthesis of PG in OA cartilage, which represents a repair effort by the chondrocytes, is suppressed by salicylate to a much greater extent than that in normal cartilage.

While the potential implications of the above studies are obvious, prediction of the *in vivo* effects of an NSAID based on its *in vitro* effects is naive. *In vitro* studies cannot predict the relative importance of the effect of an NSAID on synovitis, its direct effect on chondrocyte metabolism or its analgesic action – perhaps resulting in overloading of the damaged joint.

NSAIDs that are specific inhibitors of COX-2

Recognition that inhibition of prostaglandin synthesis by aspirin and other NSAIDs resulted in analgesic, anti-inflammatory and antipyretic effects was followed by the recognition that inhibition of the enzyme cyclo-oxygenase (COX) was responsible also for the adverse effects of these drugs. Only recently, as discussed below, has it become apparent that two isoforms of COX exist and it has become possible pharmacologically to inhibit the inducible COX isoform, whose activity results in signs of inflammation, without inhibiting the constitutive isoform, the absence of whose activity

Figure 8 Mechanism of specific COX-2 inhibition. Nonselective NSAIDs bind to the arginine at position 120 in the channel leading to the catalytic site in both COX-1 and COX-2. Therefore, they block the entrance of arachidonic acid to the catalytic site and, consequently, the production of prostaglandins, by both COX-1 and COX-2. The specificity of drugs which are specific COX-2 inhibitors (i.e. COX-1-sparing) is attributable to a single amino acid difference between the two isoenzymes at position 523, a site near arginine 120. In COX-1, position 523 is occupied by an isoleucine molecule. In COX-2, the isoleucine is replaced by a valine, which is smaller than isoleucine by a methyl group. This creates a side-pocket in the COX-2 channel, with a binding site that does not exist in COX-1. COX-2 specific agents appear to bind to the enzyme at this site, preventing arachidonic acid from reaching the catalytic site. As a result, they block the transformation of arachidonic acid to PGE$_2$ and other prostaglandins involved in pain, fever and the inflammatory response. In contrast, because COX-2 specific inhibitors are unable to bind to COX-1, prostaglandins synthesized by COX-1 which are involved in normal physiologic processes, such as protection of the GI mucosa and platelet aggregation, are not inhibited. From Hochberg MC, Katz WA, eds. *Cyclooxygenase-2 Specific Inhibition in Arthritis Therapy*. New York, NY: Center for Healthcare Education, 1999. The figure is adapted from Hawkey CJ. COX-2 inhibitors. *Lancet* 1999;353:307–14. © *The Lancet* Ltd, 1999

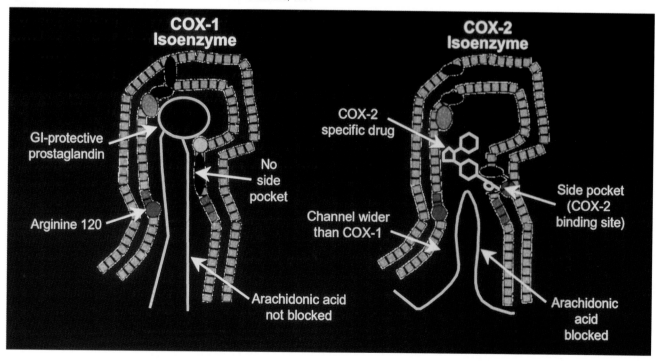

can be associated with serious and even fatal adverse effects.

COX, which is also called prostaglandin H-synthase (PGHS), catalyzes conversion of arachidonic acid to PGG_2 and then to PGH_2. Activities of a variety of other specific enzymes then produce a spectrum of arachidonic acid metabolites, including platelet-derived thromboxane ($TBXA_2$), endothelial cell-derived prostacyclin (PGI_2) and prostaglandins. Discovery in the late 1980s that COX expression in fibroblasts and monocytes could be markedly stimulated by interleukin-1 and inhibited by corticosteroids was of notable importance insofar as it had been previously thought that the level of prostaglandin production was determined only by availability of the arachidonic acid substrate. This observation led to the identification of two distinct COX isoforms, one constitutive and the other inducible (Figures 8 and 9). Separate genes for the two enzymes have since been cloned and the regulation and expression of the two proteins clarified, providing insight into their distinct biologic roles.

Concerns about the gastroenteropathy associated with nonselective NSAIDs (see above) are likely to be reduced considerably by the availability of specific COX-2 inhibitors, such as celecoxib and rofecoxib (Figure 10), both of which appear to be comparable in efficacy to – although not more effective than – nonselective NSAIDs. The advantage of

Figure 9 X-ray crystallography shows that the channel housing the catalytic site of COX-2 allows it to accept a broader range of substrates than the channel of COX-1. The tertiary structures of the COX-1 and COX-2 isoforms are virtually identical. At the catalytic site, they are completely identical with but one exception: in COX-2, the isoleucine at position 523 is replaced by valine, which is smaller than isoleucine by a single methyl group. The presence of the smaller valine creates a side-pocket in the COX-2 channel that serves as a binding site which does not exist in COX-1. COX-2 specific inhibitors bind to the enzyme at this locus. Structural modification of an NSAID by addition of a sulfonyl, sulfone or sulfonamide group provides a rigid side-extension which can enter the COX-2 side-pocket but is too bulky to fit within the COX-1 channel. On this basis, inhibitors have been developed that block the activity of COX-2 at concentrations which have only minimal effect on COX-1. On the left side of the figure, the nonselective NSAID, flurbiprofen is shown at the active site of COX-1. On the right, a prototype of celecoxib is shown at the active site of COX-2, occupying the side-pocket of the COX-2 channel. From *Evolution in Arthritis Management. Focus on Celecoxib*. Scientific Frontiers, Inc. Washington Crossing, PA., Copyright 1999 by Searle and Pfizer, Inc. The figure is reprinted with permission from data in Picot D, Loll PJ, Garavito M. The X-ray crystal structure of the membrane protein prostaglandin H_2 synthase-1. *Nature* 1994;367:243–9 and Kurumbail RG, *et al*. Structural basis for selective inhibition of cyclooxygenase-2 by anti-inflammatory agents. *Nature* 1996;384:644–8. Erratum: *Nature* 1997;385:555

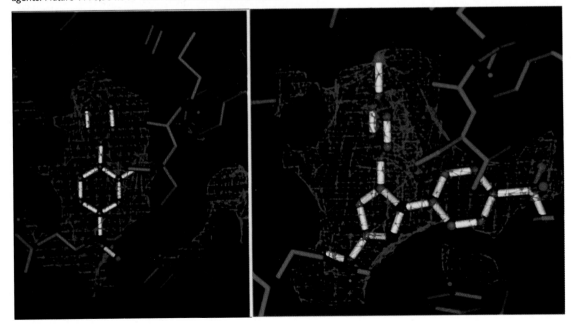

specific COX-2 inhibitors resides not in their ability to inhibit COX-2, but in their lack of inhibition of COX-1 when they are used in clinically effective doses (Table 8). Endoscopic studies have shown that the incidence of gastric and duodenal ulcers due to either of these drugs is lower than that due to comparator nonselective NSAIDs and no greater than that of placebo. Of additional advantage for the patient at risk for GI bleeding, specific COX-2 inhibitors do not affect platelet aggregation or bleeding time.

Is the striking reduction in endoscopically identifiable mucosal lesions in subjects taking specific COX-2 inhibitors accompanied by a corresponding decrease in clinically important adverse events (e.g. GI hemorrhage, perforation or obstruction)?

For patients at high risk for a serious GI complication from a nonselective NSAID, the coxibs hold an important advantage over nonselective NSAIDs. In the celecoxib long-term arthritis safety study (CLASS) – a randomized double-blinded multicenter trial in which nearly 8000 patients were treated with a supratherapeutic dose of celecoxib (400 mg bid) or with standard doses of ibuprofen (800 mg tid) or diclofenac (75 mg bid) and followed for 6 months or more – among patients who were not taking concomitant low-dose aspirin for cardiovascular prophylaxis, the annualized incidence of symptomatic ulcers and ulcer complications was significantly lower in the celecoxib group than among those taking the nonselective NSAIDs. However, the ulcer complication rate alone (i.e. excluding symptomatic ulcers) was not significantly lower than with the nonselective NSAIDs (Table 9).

Furthermore, although celecoxib use in the CLASS study was associated with a lower incidence of clinically significant decreases in hemoglobin and hematocrit, and depletion of iron stores, than the non-selective NSAID comparators, even among patients receiving low-dose aspirin, celecoxib offered no advantage with respect to the incidence of serious GI adverse events among patients also taking low-dose aspirin (some 20% of the subjects enrolled). This is relevant because the prevalence of low-dose aspirin use among patients 65 or older (an age group in which the prevalence of symptomatic OA is high) may be 50% or more.

Table 8 Classification of NSAIDs according to their selectivity in inhibiting COX-1 and COX-2

NSAID	Ratio[†]
Flurbiprofen	10.27
Ketoprofen	8.16
Fenoprofen	5.14
Tolmetin	3.93
Aspirin	3.12
Oxaprosin	2.52
Naproxen	1.79
Indomethacin	1.78
Ibuprofen	1.69
Ketorolac	1.64
Piroxicam	0.79
Nabumetone, 6-MNA	0.64
Etodolac	0.11
Celecoxib	0.11
Meloxicam	0.09
Mefenamic acid	0.08
Diclofenac	0.05
Rofecoxib	0.05
Nimesulide	0.04

[†]The ratio of the 50% inhibitory concentration (IC_{50}) of COX-2 to the IC_{50} of COX-1 in whole blood; a ratio of <1 indicates selectivity for COX-2. Modified with permission from Feldman M, McMahon AT. Do cyclooxygenase-2 inhibitors provide benefit similar to those of traditional nonsteroidal anti-inflammatory drugs, with less gastrointestinal toxicity? *Ann Intern Med* 2000;132:134–43

Figure 10 Chemical structures of celecoxib and rofecoxib

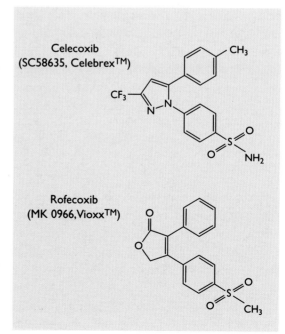

Celecoxib
(SC58635, Celebrex™)

Rofecoxib
(MK 0966, Vioxx™)

On the other hand, in the long-term GI outcome study of rofecoxib (the VIGOR study, see Table 10), in which – in contrast to the CLASS study – use of low-dose aspirin was an exclusion criterion, the incidence of myocardial infarction was some fourfold greater in the rofecoxib group than in subjects treated with the nonselective NSAID, naproxen. Whether COX-1 sparing NSAIDs, such as rofecoxib and celecoxib (perhaps by virtue of their lack of effect on platelet thromboxane synthesis with concurrent inhibition of endothelial prostacyclin production), increase the risk of thrombosis in predisposed individuals remains to be determined.

These findings are important: the benefits of low-dose aspirin for prophylaxis of cardiovascular disease are clear. Obviously, prevention of potentially fatal thromboembolic disease should take precedence over treatment of joint pain. If, as the results of the CLASS study suggest, coxibs are not more effective than non-selective NSAIDs in preventing GI catastrophes among OA patients taking low-dose aspirin, this is a significant limitation.

Homeostatic vs pro-inflammatory actions of COX-1 and COX-2

COX-1 is the only isoform expressed in normal gastric mucosa and the platelet. In the gastric antrum PGE_2 and PGI_2, synthesized as a result of the action of COX-1, promote vasodilatation, maintaining mucosal integrity. In the kidney COX-1 generates vasodilatory prostaglandins which maintain renal blood flow and glomerular filtration rate, especially in the face of systemic vasoconstriction. In platelets COX-1 is essential for the production of $TBXA_2$, which is required for platelet aggregation.

Based on the above, the concept arose that the major (if not only) function of COX-1 was to maintain homeostasis and promote specific physiologic activities. In contrast, while COX-2 was undetectable in most normal tissues, when cells such as macrophages and endothelial cells were challenged with inflammatory mediators, COX-2 expression was rapidly induced. In animal models COX-2 mRNA and protein (but not COX-1) were upregulated at sites of inflammation and detectable prior to the sharp increase in local prostaglandin production and clinical manifestations of inflammation, suggesting that COX-2 was an inducible enzyme which

accounted for a local increase in production of arachidonic acid metabolites which produced vasodilatation, edema and pain – the classical features of inflammation.

This situation is more complex, however. Studies in animals have shown that COX-2 is expressed constitutively in kidney and brain and can be induced not only by inflammation but also by physiologic stimuli in kidney, brain, ovary, uterus, cartilage and bone, while COX-1, which is constitutively present at many sites and plays a protective role, is also inducible, for example in the crypt cells of the small intestine after radiation injury, and may play a role in regeneration and contribute to inflammation. It is clear that the initial paradigm ('good' COX, 'bad' COX) is an oversimplification and that targeted pharmacologic inhibition of a specific COX-1 isoform may result in unexpected outcomes. Consideration of the role of COX-1 in several organ systems serves to emphasize this point.

Renal function

In the kidney, COX-1 is expressed in the vasculature, glomeruli and collecting ducts. It produces vasodilating prostaglandins which maintain renal plasma flow and glomerular filtration rate, especially during states of angiotensin-induced systemic vasoconstriction. Non-selective NSAIDs impair this COX-1 protective response and may result in renal ischemia, tissue damage or even papillary necrosis.

COX-2 may also be important in maintaining renal function. COX-2 knockout mice exhibit severe disruption of renal organogenesis. In the human kidney COX-2 is expressed in the podocytes of the glomerulus and endothelial cells of arteries and veins. In normal humans, specific COX-2 inhibitors induce sodium retention. This effect is associated with a marked decrease in renal PGI_2 production and is independent of any effect on renal hemodynamics. As a consequence, specific COX-2 inhibitors may cause edema and an increase in blood pressure. They are no safer than non-selective NSAIDs in this respect. Although in normal individuals, even the elderly, the glomerular filtration rate does not appear to depend on renal COX-2 activity, it is unclear whether this is true also in those with intrinsic renal disease, hypertension or volume depletion.

Table 9 Annualized incidence of upper gastrointestinal tract ulcer complications alone and with symptomatic gastroduodenal ulcers in the CLASS trial. Events/patient-years of exposure

| | Ulcer complications alone | | | Ulcer complications + symptomatic ulcers | | |
| | Treatment group | | | Treatment group | | |
	Celecoxib	NSAID	p	Celecoxib	NSAID	p
Patients not taking aspirin	5/1143	14/1101	0.04	16/1143	32/1101	0.02
Patients taking aspirin	6/298	6/283	0.92	14/298	17/283	0.49

Data from Silverstein FE, Faich G, Goldstein JL, *et al.* Gastrointestinal toxicity with celecoxib vs nonsteroidal anti-inflammatory drugs for osteoarthritis and rheumatoid arthritis. The CLASS study: a randomized controlled trial. Celecoxib Long-term Arthritis Safety Study. *JAMA* 2000;284:1247–55

Table 10 Incidence of gastrointestinal (GI) events in the VIGOR study

| Type of event | Treatment group | | Relative risk (95% CI)* | p |
| | Rofecoxib (n = 4047) | Naproxen (n = 4029) | | |
	Rate/100 patient-years			
Confirmed upper GI events	2.1	4.5	0.5 (0.3–0.6)	<0.001
Complicated confirmed upper GI events	0.6	1.4	0.4 (0.2–0.8)	0.005
Confirmed and unconfirmed upper GI events†	2.2	4.9	0.4 (0.3–0.6)	<0.001
Complicated confirmed and unconfirmed upper GI events††	0.6	1.6	0.4 (0.2–0.7)	0.002
All episodes of GI bleeding	1.1	3.0	0.4 (0.3–0.6)	<0.001

*Gastroduodenal perforation or obstruction, upper gastrointestinal bleeding or symptomatic gastroduodenal ulcer. †The analysis includes 13 events reported by investigators but considered to be unconfirmed by the end-point committee. ††The analysis includes six events reported by investigators but considered to be unconfirmed by the end-point committee. Modified from Bombardier C, Laine L, Reicin A, *et al.* Comparison of upper gastrointestinal toxicity of rofecoxib amd naproxen in patients with rheumatoid arthritis. *N Engl J Med* 2000;343:1520–28

Gastrointestinal tract

COX-1 is the only COX isoform in the gastric mucosa and protects the stomach from erosions and ulceration. Gastrointestinal bleeding caused by non-specific NSAIDs appears to relate to their inhibition of COX-1 activity both in the platelet, increasing the tendency to bleed, and in the gastric mucosa, increasing the likelihood of ulceration. Because COX-2 is not present in normal gastric mucosa or the platelet, it might be expected that inhibition would impose no risk of gastric ulceration or bleeding. However, COX-2 is expressed in animal models with acute gastric erosion and ulceration and may play a role in facilitating ulcer healing. Similarly, in humans COX-2 is induced with gastric injury and can be demonstrated at the rim of gastric ulcers. Furthermore, COX-2 inhibitors retard ulcer healing in animals. Whether healing of NSAID-induced ulcers will be impaired in patients who are switched from a non-selective NSAID to a COX-2 inhibitor is uncertain. It has been suggested that specific COX-2

inhibitors will increase the risk of major GI adverse effects by retarding the healing of ulcers induced by other stimuli, e.g. *H. pylori* or concomitant aspirin use. The clinical impact, if any, of specific COX-2 inhibition under these circumstances has not been established and the relative risk of GI bleeding associated with specific COX-2 inhibitors is uncertain.

Might COX-2 inhibitors cause ulcers in predisposed individuals? Patients with erosions or a history of ulcer are more likely to develop ulcers than those without erosions or ulcer history, probably because of reactivation of damage at the site of the ulcer scar. Because it is likely that COX-2 is induced in both of these situations, it remains to be shown that specific COX-2 inhibitors will not increase ulcer risk in these subgroups.

COX-2 may also play an important physiologic role in other parts of the GI tract. COX-2 levels are increased in inflammatory bowel disease, such as ulcerative colitis, and selective inhibition of COX-2 has been shown to exacerbate inflammation in an

Table 11 Selected gastrointestinal symptoms in pooled Celecoxib and Rofecoxib trials

Drug	Symptom	Subjects receiving placebo (% with complaint)	Subjects receiving COX-2 inhibitor (% with complaint)	Subjects receiving ibuprofen (2400 mg/d) (% with complaint)	Subjects receiving diclofenac (150 mg/d) (% with complaint)
Celecoxib[†]	Abdominal pain	2.8	4.1	9.0	9.0
(200–400 mg/d)	Dyspepsia	6.2	8.8	10.9	12.8
	Nausea	4.2	3.5	3.4	6.7
	Diarrhea	3.8	5.6	9.3	5.8
Rofecoxib[‡]	Abdominal pain	4.1	3.4	4.6	5.8
(12–25 mg/d)	Dyspepsia	2.7	3.5	4.7	4.0
	Nausea	4.7	5.2	7.1	7.4
	Diarrhea	6.8	6.5	7.1	10.6

[†]Trials involved a total of 8108 patients. Withdrawals due to adverse events occurred in 7.1% of celecoxib-treated patients in controlled celecoxib trials and in 6.1% of placebo recipients. Withdrawal due to abdominal pain or dyspepsia occurred in 0.7% and 0.8% of celecoxib-treated patients and in 0.6% and 0.6% of placebo recipients, respectively. [‡]Trials involved a total of 4957 patients. No published information is available on withdrawal rates. From Feldman M, McMahon T. Do cyclooxygenase-2 inhibitors provide benefits similar to those of traditional nonsteroidal anti-inflammatory drugs with less gastrointestinal toxicity? *Ann Intern Med* 2000;132:134–43

Figure 11 Percentage change in number of colorectal polyps at 6 months (individual patient data and mean values) in patients taking celecoxib; *p = 0.003 vs placebo. Modified from Slide Kit FAP (Familial Adenomatous Polyposis): A New Indication for CELEBREX® (celecoxib capsules). Searle/Pfizer. © 2000; 3/00, YCE18652U

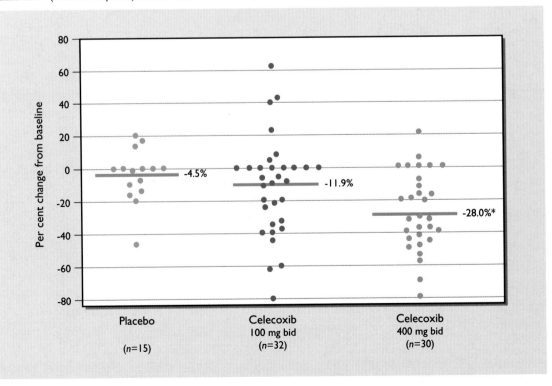

animal model of colitis. It remains to be seen whether specific COX-2 inhibitors are safe in humans with ulcerative colitis.

Are specific COX-2 inhibitors superior to non-selective NSAIDs with regard to nonspecific GI complaints? In an analysis of eight previously published double-blind randomized trials which varied among themselves with respect to treatment duration, comparator NSAIDs and inclusion of a placebo group, the cumulative incidence of non-specific GI adverse events (e.g. dyspepsia) was slightly lower with rofecoxib than with nonselective NSAIDs over a 6-month treatment period (23.5% vs 25.5%, $p=0.02$), but was no better than that with nonselective NSAIDs thereafter (Table 11). Celecoxib and non-selective NSAIDs were both associated with more abdominal pain, dyspepsia and diarrhea than placebo. However, use of celecoxib was accompanied by less abdominal pain than was seen with ibuprofen, diclofenac or naproxen, and less dyspepsia than with naproxen. In general, non-specific GI symptoms caused by rofecoxib did not differ from those caused by placebo or comparator NSAID, except that diarrhea was more common with diclofenac than with rofecoxib.

Ovarian and uterine function

COX-2 mediated prostaglandin production is associated with parturition and is implicated also in ovulation, fertilization and implantation. COX-2 is induced immediately after the surge of luteinizing hormone and seems necessary for production of the proteolytic enzymes required for rupture of the ovarian follicle. Inhibition of follicular rupture may explain the infertility associated with NSAID use.

Thrombosis

Maintenance of normal blood flow and generation of an appropriate thrombogenic response to injury require a delicate balance between the activities of $TBXA_2$ produced by platelets, and PGI_2 from vascular endothelial cells (Table 12). Activated platelets generate $TBXA_2$ via the action of COX-1. Platelet aggregation results in the release of $TBXA_2$, which then provides a substrate and stimulus for production by vascular endothelial cells of PGI_2, a potent vasodilator which counteracts the vasoconstrictive action of $TBXA_2$. It has been shown that shear stress

Table 12 Cyclo-oxygenase activity and thrombosis

	Platelet	Endothelial cell
Cyclo-oxygenase isoform	COX-1	COX-2
Active arachidonic acid metabolite	Thromboxane A_2	Prostacyclin
Function of isoform	Activates fibrinogen receptors	Inhibits platelet function
	Induces vasoconstriction	Stimulates smooth muscle relaxation and vasodilation

induces COX-2 expression in endothelial cells, leading to production of substantial amounts of PGI_2 by these cells. It appears that a substantial proportion of systemic PGI_2 production is derived from the action of COX-2.

In humans, PGI_2 production can be inhibited by specific COX-2 inhibitors. Because nonselective NSAIDs inhibit both COX-1 and COX-2, their effects on pro- and anti-thrombotic activities are presumably in balance. However, specific COX-2 inhibitors may limit production of PGI_2 by endothelial cells, while having no effect on $TBXA_2$ production by platelets. This could theoretically result in an imbalance favoring platelet aggregation and vaso-constriction, with an increase in the frequency of vascular occlusion. Whether this is a clinically important effect of specific COX-2 inhibition remains to be determined, especially in patients at risk for ischemic events. The question is important, since deaths from cardiovascular disease far outnumber those from NSAID-induced gastropathy.

Neoplasia and Alzheimer's disease

Recent work has delineated a role for COX-2 in the development and progression of adenomatous polyps and carcinoma of the colon, and in the progression of Alzheimer's disease. Recent data indicate that treatment with celecoxib, 400 mg/bid, significantly reduced the number of colorectal polyps by nearly 30%, in comparison with placebo ($p = 0.003$) in a 6-month trial in patients with familial adenomatous polyposis. The effect of COX-2 inhibition on the development of colorectal cancer in patients with familial or non-familial adenomatous polyps has not been established (Figure 11).

Bibliography

American College of Rheumatology Subcommittee on Osteoarthritis Guidelines. Recommendations for the medical management of osteoarthritis of the hip and knee: 2000 update. *Arthritis Rheum* 2000;43:1905–15

Beard K, Walker AM, Perera DR, *et al.* Nonsteroidal anti-inflammatory drugs and hospitalization for gastroesophageal bleeding in the elderly. *Arch Intern Med* 1987;47:1621–3

Bombardier C, Laine L, Reicin A, *et al.* Comparison of upper gastrointestinal toxicity of rofecoxib and naproxen in patients with rheumatoid arthritis. *N Engl J Med* 2000;343:1520–28

Bradley J, Katz BP, Brandt KD. Severity of knee pain does not predict a better response to an anti-inflammatory dose of ibuprofen than to analgesic therapy in patients with osteoarthritis. *J Rheumatol* 2001: in press

Bradley JD, Brandt KD, Katz BP, *et al.* Comparison of an anti-inflammatory dose of ibuprofen, an analgesic dose of ibuprofen, and acetaminophen in the treatment of patients with osteoarthritis of the knee. *N Engl J Med* 1991;325:87–91

Celecoxib for arthritis. *The Medical Letter* 1999;41: 11–12

Crofford L. COX-1 and COX-2 tissue expression: implications and predictions. *J Rheumatol* 1997;24:15–19

Crofford LJ, Oates JC, McCune WJ, *et al.* Thrombosis in patients with connective tissue diseases treated with specific cyclooxygenase 2 inhibitors. *Arthritis Rheum* 2000;43:1891–96

Dieppe P, Cushnaghan J, Jasani MK, *et al.* A 2-year, placebo controlled trial of nonsteroidal anti-inflammatory therapy in osteoarthritis of the knee joint. *Br J Rheumatol* 1993;32:595–600

Dubois RN, Abramson SB, Crofford L, *et al.* Cyclooxygenase in biology and disease. *FASEB J* 1998;1063–73

Fries JF, Miller SR, Spitz PW, *et al.* Towards an epidemiology of gastropathy associated with nonsteroidal anti-inflammatory drug use. *Gastroenterology* 1989;96:647–55

Goldstein JL. Celecoxib is associated with reduced chronic gastrointestinal (GI) blood loss relative to nonsteroidal anti-inflammatory drugs (NSAIDs). *Arthritis Rheum* 2000;43(Suppl 9)S147:482

Griffin MR, Piper JM, Daughtery JR, *et al.* Nonsteroidal anti-inflammatory drug use and increased risk for peptic ulcer disease in elderly persons. *Ann Intern Med* 1991;114:257–63

Hawkey CJ, Karrasch JA, Szczepanski L, *et al.* Omeprazole compared with misoprostol for ulcers associated with nonsteroidal anti-inflammatory drugs. *N Engl J Med* 1998;338:727–34

Heerdink ER, Leufkens HG, Herings MC, *et al.* NSAIDs associated with increased risk of congestive heart failure in elderly patients taking diuretics. *Arch Intern Med* 1998;158:1108–12

Henrich WL, Agodoa LE, Barrett B, *et al.* Analgesics and the kidney: summary and recommendations to the Scientific Advisory Board of the National Kidney Foundation from an ad hoc committee of the National Kidney Foundation. *Am J Kidney Dis* 1996;27:162–5

Hochberg MC, Altman RD, Brandt KD, *et al.* Guidelines for the medical management of osteoarthritis. Part I. Osteoarthritis of the hip. *Arthritis Rheum* 1995;38: 1535–40

Hochberg MC, Altman RD, Brandt KD, *et al.* Guidelines for the medical management of osteoarthritis. Part II. Osteoarthritis of the knee. *Arthritis Rheum* 1995;38: 1541–6

McLaughlin J, Seth R, Cole AT, *et al.* Increased inducible cyclo-oxygenase associated with treatment failure in ulcerative colitis. *Gastroenterology* 1966;110:A964

Miettinen S, Fusco F, Yrjanheikki J, *et al.* Spreading depression and focal brain ischemia induce cyclo-oxygenase-2 in cortical neurons through N-methyl-D-aspartic acid-receptors and phospholipase A2. *Proc Natl Acad Sci (USA)* 1997;94:6500–5

Raskin JB, White RH, Jackson JE, *et al.* Misoprostol dosage in the prevention of nonsteroidal anti-inflammatory drug-induced gastric and duodenal ulcers: a comparison of three regimens. *Ann Intern Med* 1995;123:344–50

Scheiman JM. NSAIDs, gastrointestinal injury, and cytoprotection. *Gastro Clin N Am* 1996;25:279–99

Scholes D, Stergachis A, Penna PM, *et al.* Nonsteroidal antiinflammatory drug discontinuation in patients with osteoarthritis. *J Rheumatol* 1995;22:708–12

Silverstein FE, Graham DY, Senior JR, *et al.* Misoprostol reduces serious gastrointestinal complications in patients with rheumatoid arthritis receiving nonsteroidal anti-inflammatory drugs: a randomized, double-blind, placebo-controlled trial. *Ann Intern Med* 1995;123:241–9

Silverstein FE, Faich G, Goldstein JL, *et al.* Gastro-intestinal toxicity with celecoxib vs nonsteroidal anti-inflammatory drugs for osteoarthritis and rheumatoid arthritis. The CLASS study: a randomized controlled trial. Celecoxib Long-term Arthritis Safety Study. *JAMA* 2000;284:1247–55

Simon LS, Lanza FL, Lipsky PE, *et al.* Preliminary study of the safety and efficacy of SC-58365, a novel cyclo-oxygenase 2 inhibitor. *Arthritis Rheum* 1998;41:1591–602

Somerville K, Faulkner G, Langman M. Nonsteroidal anti-inflammatory drugs and bleeding peptic ulcer. *Lancet* 1986;1:462–4

Steward WF, Kawas C, Corrado M, Metter EJ. Risk of Alzheimer's disease and duration of NSAID use. *Neurology* 1997;48:626–32

Vane JR, Botting RM. Mechanism of action of aspirin-like drugs. *Semin Arthritis Rheum* 1997;26:2–10

Wolfe F, Zhao S, Lane N. Preference for non-steroidal anti-inflammatory drugs (NSAIDs) over acetaminophen by rheumatic disease patients: a survey of 1799 patients with osteoarthritis, rheumatoid arthritis and fibromyalgia. *Arthritis Rheum* 2000;43:378–85

Wolfe MM, Lichtenstein DR, Singh G. Gastrointestinal toxicity of nonsteroidal anti- inflammatory drugs. *New Engl J Med* 1999;340:1888–99

Yeomans NE, Tulassay Z, Juhasz L, *et al.* A comparison of omeprazole with ranitidine for ulcers associated with nonsteroidal anti-inflammatory drugs. *N Engl J Med* 1998;338:719–26

CHAPTER ELEVEN

Systemic pharmacologic therapy

II. Opioids in the treatment of osteoarthritis

In general, chronic opioid therapy has had little place in the management of chronic osteoarthritis pain. Side-effects of opioids that may be especially problematic in the elderly include: nausea, vomiting, constipation, urinary retention, mental confusion, drowsiness and respiratory depression. Among patients who have chronic obstructive pulmonary disease or decreased respiratory reserve, depression of the respiratory drive may occur even with a low dose of opioid. Furthermore, although the elderly patient without pulmonary disease who takes an opioid chronically is often tolerant of the respiratory depressant effect of opioids, the addition of a general anesthetic, sedative-hypnotic or other central nervous system depressant will increase the risk.

The central nervous system effects of opioids (for example dizziness) may have particularly serious consequences in the elderly. Elderly persons for whom either codeine or propoxyphene were prescribed were found to have a relative risk of hip fracture of 1.6 (95% CI, 1.4–1.9). Concurrent use of these opioids and a psychotropic drug (e.g. sedative, antidepressant or antipsychotic) carried a fracture risk of 2.6 (95% CI, 2.0–3.4) times that of nonusers of either drug class.

In addition to their concerns about side-effects, health professionals and patients hold concerns related to tolerance to opioids and physical and psychologic dependence. Many physicians are reluctant to prescribe opioids for patients with nonmalignant chronic pain because of their concerns about legal action by governmental regulatory agencies. More recent evidence, however, suggests that the prohibition of opioids on these grounds may require re-evaluation. The desire to reduce illicit drug use in society may exaggerate fears of drug dependency and addiction. In fact, people aged 60 or older account for fewer than 1% of patients attending methadone maintenance programs, suggesting that the prevalence of narcotic abuse among older people is low. Table 1 provides a list of signs which are suggestive of opioid addiction.

The dose of opioid analgesic medication needed to treat chronic nonmalignant pain, such as OA pain, is often lower than that needed for cancer-related pain. If opioid treatment is started with a low dose which is then increased gradually, serious side-effects, such as impaired consciousness and respiratory suppression, are rare. With chronic use tolerance to opioids is common. The patient first notices a shorter duration of analgesia and then a

Table I. Signs suggestive of addiction in patients taking an opioid for pain*

Loss of control
- Compulsive overuse, unable to take medications as prescribed
- Frequently runs out of medication early despite dose agreement
- Frequently reports lost or stolen prescriptions
- Solicits multiple prescribers
- Uses multiple pharmacies to fill prescriptions

Preoccupation with drug use
- Noncompliant with other treatment recommendations
- Misses other appointments, always arrives for opioid prescriptions
- Uses street drugs, involved with street culture
- Preference for short-acting or bolus dose medications
- Reports no relief with other medications or treatments
- Reports allergies to all other drugs

Adverse consequences of opioid use
- Declining function despite apparent analgesia
- Observed to be frequently intoxicated or high
- Persistently oversedated

*Occasional occurrences may be understandable in the context of pain alone. However, a persistent pattern of behavior should raise concern regarding possible addiction. Reproduced with permission from Savage SR. Opioid use in the management of chronic pain. *Med Clin North Am* 1999;83:761–86

decrease in the effectiveness of each dose. Tolerance can be delayed by using low doses and concomitantly administering a non-opioid analgesic. Notably, tolerance to most of the adverse effects of opioids, including respiratory and central nervous system depression, develops as rapidly as, or more rapidly than, tolerance to their analgesic action so that adequate analgesia can be restored safely by increasing the dose.

What about the efficacy of commonly used opioids? Oral codeine, when taken alone in a dose of 60 mg, is no more effective than 650 mg of aspirin or acetaminophen. Codeine, therefore, is usually used in combination with these drugs to treat moderate or moderately severe pain. Although the codeine congener, propoxyphene, which is available as 65 mg of the hydrochloride or 100 mg of the napsylate, is no more effective than 32 mg of codeine or aspirin or acetaminophen, formulations of propoxyphene in combination with acetaminophen or aspirin are more effective than propoxyphene alone.

Opioid analgesics deserve consideration for acute flares of joint pain when acetaminophen or an NSAID do not produce adequate analgesia or when the patient is unable to tolerate NSAIDs. The effective dose varies widely from patient to patient. If an opioid is necessary for treatment of chronic joint pain in the patient with OA, once the optimal dose needed to provide adequate analgesia (preferably for at least 4 hours) has been established by titration, the drug should generally be given on a fixed schedule, with the patient informed that he may omit a dose if he is not in pain. Around-the-clock administration is more effective than waiting for severe pain to return before administering the next dose and may decrease the total dose required. It should be emphasized, however, that in most patients with OA for whom an opioid is prescribed, joint pain is not constant and non-opioid analgesics, NSAIDs and nonpharmacologic measures are effective in combating joint pain and permitting reduction in the dose of opioid. Indeed, in most patients with OA, such measures obviate the need for opioid therapy.

Tramadol hydrochloride is a centrally acting analgesic that binds with a dual mechanism of action: the molecule is a μ-opioid agonist and inhibits the re-uptake of norepinephrine and serotonin. The affinity of binding to the μ-opioid regimen is some 6000 times lower than that of morphine. Because its opioid and nonopioid activities are synergistic, the analgesic effect of tramadol is only partly antagonized by naloxone. Tramadol does not inhibit prostaglandin synthesis and hence, in contrast to NSAIDs, has no adverse effects on the kidney, platelet or gastric mucosa.

Oral administration of tramadol may be useful in the management of moderate to moderately severe pain. In a dose of 300 mg/d, tramadol was more effective than 300 mg/d of dextropropoxyphene. A dose of 100 mg has been shown to be more effective than 60 mg of codeine and about as

Table 2 Pretreatment pain intensity and total pain relief scores for efficacy evaluations in elderly patients with chronic pain

Measurements	Tramadol*			Acetaminophen/codeine[†]		
	n	Mean score	95% CI	n	Mean score	95% CI
Pretreatment pain intensity**						
Day1, week 1	224	2.2	2.1–2.3	150	2.3	2.2–2.4
Day week 3	170	2.0	1.9–2.1	113	2.0	1.9–2.2
Total pain relief[††]						
Day 1, week 1	221	6.1	5.6–6.6	147	6.1	5.4–6.7
Day1, week 3	169	7.4	6.8–7.9	111	6.7	6.0–7.4

CI, confidence interval; *Maximum daily dose, 400 mg; [†]Maximum daily dose, 2400 mg acetaminophen/240 mg codeine; **Scale: 0 = none, 1 = mild, 2 = moderate, 3 = severe; [††]Scale: 0 = no relief, 16 = complete relief at every evaluation. Reprinted by permission of the publisher from Rauck RL, Ruoff GE, McMillen JI. Comparison of tramadol and acetaminophen with codeine for long-term pain management in elderly patients. *Curr Ther Res* 1994;55:1417–31 © Excerpta Medica Inc.

Figure 1 Pain scores, in cm, measured on a 10 cm visual analog scale (VAS), at the intervals depicted in a 39-day trial in which patients with knee osteoarthritis received tramadol, 200–400 mg/day, or ibuprofen 1200–2400 mg/day. Improvement in knee pain in the two treatment groups was comparable. Reproduced with permission from Katz WB. Progress with tramadol: US experience. *Clin Courier* 1997;14:1–12

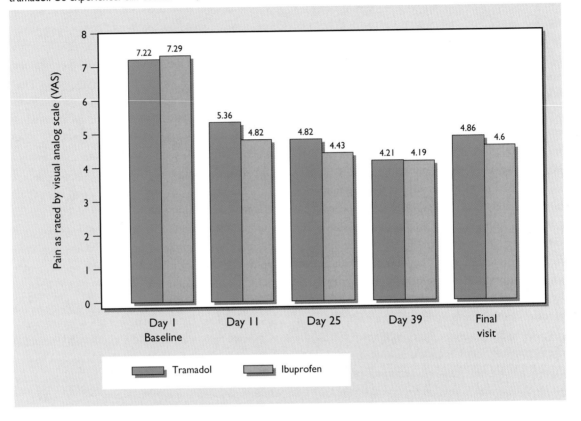

Table 3 Mean minimum effective daily naproxen dose in naproxen responders and nonresponders being treated with tramadol or placebo

	Minimum effective daily naproxen dose (mg)	p value
Naproxen responders[†]		
Tramadol	221	0.02
Placebo	407	
Naproxen nonresponders[‡]		
Tramadol	419	NS
Placebo	396	

[†]Patients whose baseline pain score, measured on a visual analog scale (VAS) while taking naproxen 1000mg/day, was <40 mm and was ≥20mm lower than their VAS score at the end of a washout period prior to naproxen administration; [‡]patients whose baseline pain score on a VAS was ≥40mm or was <20mm lower than their VAS score at the end of a washout, prior to institution of naproxen treatment; NS, not significant. Reproduced with permission from Schnitzer TJ, Kamin M, Olson W. Tramadol allows reduction of naproxen dose among patients with naproxen-responsive osteoarthritis pain. A randomized, double-blind, placebo-controlled study. *Arthritis Rheum* 1999;42:1370–7

effective as combinations of codeine with aspirin or with acetaminophen (Table 2), which are considerably less expensive. In a randomized double-blinded parallel study of subjects with chronic joint pain, tramadol 200–400 mg/day produced a level of improvement to that seen with ibuprofen 1200–2400 mg/day (Figure 1). Tramadol was reported to be a useful adjunct in patients with OA at a variety of joint sites whose symptoms were inadequately controlled with NSAIDs. In a placebo-controlled trial which was confined to patients with knee OA who demonstrated an ability to tolerate tramadol in an initial 'run-in' phase of the study, among those whose joint pain improved with naproxen 1000 mg/d the addition of tramadol permitted a reduction in the dose of NSAID without compromising pain-relief – i.e. tramadol was NSAID-sparing (Table 3).

However tramadol may have significant side-effects. In a 4-week clinical trial comparing tramadol with an acetaminophen/codeine combination, nausea was significantly more common with tramadol (10.3% *vs* 4.5%; $p \geq 0.05$). Central nervous system side-effects (e.g. dizziness, vertigo, somnolence) also were more common with tramadol, although these differences were not significant. Adverse events considered by the investigators as being probably related to treatment occurred in 17% of those in the tramadol group and 12.2% in the paracetamol/codeine group, but led to discontinuation of treatment in twice as many patients taking tramadol as paracetamol/codeine (18.8% *vs* 9.6%, respectively; $p < 0.05$).

The frequency and severity of side-effects of tramadol may be reduced considerably if treatment is initiated at a very low dose (e.g. 25 mg/day), which can then be increased gradually every few days. (This 'go slow' approach, however, limits the usefulness of the drug in the management of acute pain.) The development of tolerance or dependence with long-term administration of tramadol appears to be uncommon. Accordingly, even though it has some opioid activity, tramadol has not been scheduled as a controlled substance. The rate of abuse/dependence among tramadol users was found to be 1.55 cases per 100 000 individuals exposed. Among those who abused tramadol, 97% had a prior history of substance abuse.

Because it inhibits re-uptake of serotonin and norepinephrine, tramadol should not generally be given to patients who are receiving a tricyclic antidepressant, selective serotonin re-uptake inhibitor or monoamine oxidase inhibitor. The combination has been reported to cause convulsions. Even in the absence of concomitant therapy with the above agents, seizures may occur in some patients taking tramadol; the risk is greater in patients with a prior history of seizures.

Tramadol may be particularly useful for treatment of OA pain in patients in whom acetaminophen or a low dose of NSAID is ineffective or in whom contraindications exist to the use of an NSAID, for example a prior history of NSAID-induced gastrointestinal bleeding or impairment of renal function. In such patients a trial of tramadol may be preferable to a high dose of a nonspecific COX-2 inhibitor.

Bibliography

Caldwell JR, Hale ME, Boyd RE, *et al.* Treatment of osteoarthritis pain with controlled release oxycodone or fixed combination oxycodone plus acetaminophen added to nonsteroidal anti-inflammatory drugs: a double blind, randomized, multicenter, placebo controlled trial. *J Rheumatol* 1999;26:862–9

Foley KM. Changing concepts of tolerance to opioids. What the cancer patient has taught us. In Chapman CR, Foley KM, eds. *Current and Emerging Issues in Cancer Pain: Research and Practice*. New York: Raven Press; 1993:331–50

Raffa RB, Friderichs E, Reimann W, *et al.* Opioid and nonopioid components independently contribute to the mechanism of action of tramadol, an 'atypical' opioid analgesic. *J Pharmacol Exp Ther* 1992;260: 275–85

Rauck RL, Ruoff GE, McMillen JI. Comparison of tramadol and acetaminophen with codeine for long-term pain management in elderly patients. *Curr Ther Res* 1994;55:1417–31

Schnitzer TJ, Kamin M, Olson W. Tramadol allows reduction of naproxen dose among patients with naproxen-responsive osteoarthritis pain. A randomized, double-blind, placebo-controlled study. *Arthritis Rheum* 1999;42:1370–7

Shorr RI, Griffin MR, Daugherty JR, Ray WA. Opioid analgesics and the risk of hip fracture in the elderly: codeine and propoxyphene. *J Gerontol* 1992;47(4):M111–15

CHAPTER TWELVE

Local therapy for OA pain

1. Rubefacients and capsaicin cream

Although NSAIDs and analgesics such as aceta-minophen are the agents most commonly used to control the pain of osteoarthritis, they often produce no more than a moderate reduction in joint pain and their use, especially in the elderly, is often attended by side-effects such as dyspepsia, gastrointestinal bleeding and renal dysfunction. Furthermore, older individuals with OA often require systemic medication for comorbid conditions (e.g. hypertension, heart disease, diabetes mellitus), increasing the risk of serious drug interactions with NSAIDs and compounding the problem of compliance with prescribed dosing. For this reason, management of OA pain by topical therapy holds considerable appeal.

Application of topical irritants to painful joints and muscles and the local heat provided by rubefacients may be beneficial. However, although topical medications are widely used in the United States as over-the-counter preparations, they are not often prescribed for OA by physicians in that country, chiefly because evidence of their efficacy is limited. Topical NSAIDs, in particular, enjoy considerable popularity in Europe, but have not been approved for use in the United States. It is unclear whether the benefit attributed to their use is mediated through a pharmacologic action, placebo effect or through their action as a rubefacient. On the other hand, in contrast to the uncertainties surrounding the use of topical NSAIDs, controlled clinical trials indicate that topically applied capsaicin cream may relieve joint pain in patients with OA of the hand or knee.

Capsaicin (8-methyl-N-vanillyl-6-nonenamide) (Figure 1) is an alkaloid derived from the seeds and membranes of the Nightshade family of plants, which includes the common pepper plant (Figure 2). It is the active ingredient in tabasco sauce. Initially, it was believed that capsaicin worked via a 'counter-irritant' mechanism but it was subsequently shown that when applied topically, capsaicin stimulates the release of substance P from peripheral nerves and prevents reaccumulation of substance P from cell bodies and nerve terminals in both the central and peripheral nervous systems. This action is relevant because substance P is an important neuropeptide mediator responsible for the transmission of pain from the periphery to the central nervous system. Capsaicin has been used successfully in the treatment of a variety of painful disorders, including postherpetic neuralgia, cluster headaches, diabetic neuropathy, phantom limb pain and postmastectomy pain. Because local application of capsaicin results in the depletion of substance P from the entire neuron, branches from the peripheral nerves to deeper structures, such as the joint, are effectively depleted. Initially, external transport of substance P is blocked; with continued treatment, the synthesis of substance P is reduced.

Figure 1 Capsaicin (8-methyl-N-vanillyl-6-nonenamide)

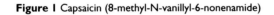

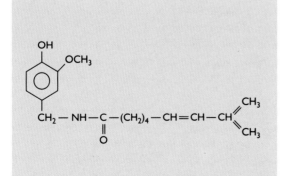

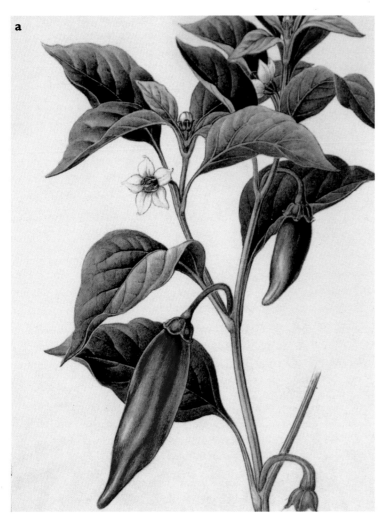

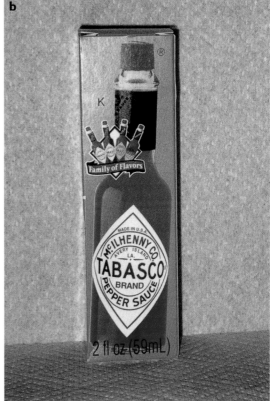

Figure 2 The fruit of the *Capsicum annuum* (a) is used as a condiment. From Bunney S. *The Illustrated Book of Herbs. Their Medicinal and Culinary Uses.* New York, NY: Gallery Books, 1985:96. Capsaicin is the major ingredient in tabasco sauce (b)

Although articular cartilage is not innervated and, therefore, cannot be a source of pain, histologic studies have shown that the joint capsule (see Figure 8 in chapter on Clinical Features), tendons, ligaments and periosteum are extensively innervated. Nerve fibers are present also in subchondral bone. Nerve fibers in synovium have been shown to localize antiserum to substance P and synovial fluid concentrations of substance P are increased in patients with OA.

In addition to modulating pain, substance P may mediate inflammation within the joint. For example, intra-articular infusion of substance P in rats with adjuvant arthritis increased the severity of joint inflammation. Intra-articular injection of substance P increases blood flow to the joint, transudation of plasma proteins and release of lysosomal enzymes. Substance P is a chemo-attractant for neutrophils and monocytes and stimulates synovial cells to produce prostaglandins and collagenase, mediators associated with joint damage. Although the importance of substance P in the pathogenesis of joint inflammation in OA is not clear, it plays a significant role in mediating joint pain in OA and its pharmacologic inhibition may be useful in the palliation of joint pain in this disease.

As shown in Table 1, several studies have demonstrated the efficacy of capsaicin cream in the treatment of OA pain. While patients in most of these clinical trials have generally been permitted to continue their usual treatment with NSAIDs or analgesics, capsaicin cream has been shown to be effective even when employed as monotherapy for OA, and improvement in pain scores under such

Table I   Results of placebo-controlled trials of capsaicin cream in patients with osteoarthritis

Reference	OA joint site	Capsaicin strength	Duration of study	Number of subjects treated	% of subjects reporting a decrease in joint pain at end of study	
					Capsaicin	Placebo
Deal et al.	Knee	0.025%	4 weeks	36 Capsaicin 34 Placebo	22%	14%
McCarthy et al.	DIP, PIP, MCP	0.075%	4 weeks	7 Capsaicin 7 Placebo	60%	20%
Altman et al.	Various (70% knee)	0.025%	12 weeks	57 Capsaicin 56 Placebo	53%	27%

DIP, distal interphalangeal joints; PIP, proximal interphalangeal joints; MCP, metacarpophalangeal joints. Reproduced from Brandt KD, Bradley JD. Topical capsaicin cream. In Brandt KD, Doherty M, Lohmander LS, eds. *Osteoarthritis*. Oxford: Oxford University Press, 1998:296–9; by permission of Oxford University Press

conditions has been shown to persist for as long as 12 weeks and to be as great as that which can be achieved with NSAIDs.

A local burning sensation is common in patients who use capsaicin preparations, but this diminishes with continued treatment and seldom results in discontinuation of the treatment. Intolerance may also be managed by temporarily switching to a lower strength preparation (if the 0.025% formulation is not the initial choice). A higher potency cream may then be used, if necessary, after tolerance to the skin irritating effect of the lower strength preparation has developed. Because burning at the application site affects blinding in clinical trials and could favor a positive response to capsaicin, it is notable that the therapeutic response among subjects who experienced burning after treatment with capsaicin was comparable to that in those who did not incur this side-effect.

Topical capsaicin therapy appears to be safe and effective and warrants initial consideration in the management of OA pain. Patients should apply the cream in a thin film to all sides of the involved joint and should be instructed to wash their hands immediately after application of the cream, and to avoid contact with broken or inflamed skin, eyes and mucus membranes.

Bibliography

Altman RD, Aven A, Holmburg, CE, et al. Capsaicin cream 0.025% as monotherapy for osteoarthritis: a double-blind study. *Semin Arthritis Rheum* 1994;23:25–33

Brandt KD, Bradley JD. Topical capsaicin cream. In Brandt KD, Doherty M, Lohmander LS, eds. *Osteoarthritis*. Oxford, UK: Oxford University Press, 1998:296–9

Deal CL, Schnitzer, TJ, Lipstein E, et al. Treatment of arthritis with topical capsaicin: a double-blind trial. *Clin Ther* 1991;13:383

Fitzgerald M. Capsaicin and sensory neurones: a review. *Pain* 1983;15:109–30

McCarthy GM, McCarty DJ. Effect of topical capsaicin in the therapy of painful osteoarthritis of the hands. *J Rheumatol* 1992;19:604

Schnitzer T, Posner M, Lawrence I. High strength capsaicin cream for osteoarthritis pain: rapid onset of action and improved efficacy with twice daily dosing. *J Clin Rheumatol* 1995;1:268–73

Virus RM, Gebhard GF. Pharmacologic actions of capsaicin: apparent involvement of substance P and serotonin. *Life Sci* 1979;25:1273–84

CHAPTER TWELVE

Local therapy for OA pain

II. Intra-articular corticosteroid injection

Systemic corticosteroid treatment or administration of adrenocorticotropic hormone has no place in the treatment of osteoarthritis. The beneficial effects are equivocal and the side-effects associated with prolonged use of these agents, especially in the elderly, far outweigh any possible efficacy. On the other hand, intra-articular injection of corticosteroids may be of benefit in OA, although symptomatic improvement is likely to be only temporary (Figure 1). The data indicate that intra-articular injection of glucocorticoid appears to produce greater symptomatic benefit than injection of placebo for a couple of weeks, perhaps, but does not afford benefit of longer duration.

Pain relief after intra-articular steroid injection in OA may be associated with a decrease in synovial permeability, even when the drug produces an increase in synovial fluid leukocytosis as a result of synovitis generated by the microcrystalline formulation (Figure 2). Furthermore, steroids inhibit hyaluronic acid secretion by the synovium, which may help to decrease the volume of synovial effusion.

The adverse effects of corticosteroid injections are generally relatively minor but some, such as atrophy of skin and subcutaneous fat (Figures 3 and 4), may result in litigation. This complication results in a depressed, atrophic area which is often made more obvious by associated hypopigmentation. Factors associated with development of atrophy include poor localization of the injection and use of potent fluorinated steroids. It is prudent to warn patients of the possibility of cutaneous or subcutaneous atrophy when injecting superficial sites, such as the acromioclavicular joint or the small joints of the hands, and to document this discussion in the medical record. In addition, injection

of fluorinated steroids should be avoided at these sites.

Although temporary deterioration in diabetes control might be expected owing to systemic absorption of corticosteroid, it is not common. Nonetheless, it is best to warn patients of the possibility. In some patients, facial flushing occurs after an intra-articular corticosteroid injection. The incidence of flushing is unclear, but one prospective study has suggested that it may be as high as 40%, and may be severe in 12%. Changing to a different corticosteroid may reduce the risk of subsequent flushing. Anaphylaxis has been reported after corticosteroid injection but is rare.

Sepsis is the most worrysome complication of intra-articular steroid injection, and may result in severe morbidity and significant mortality. Infection may be a complication of any intra-articular puncture, but many consider that the risk is greater in the presence of corticosteroids. The true risk of joint infection following corticosteroid injection is unknown. Most estimates are derived from retrospective records and are of the order of 1 per 15000 to 1 per 50000 injections. Clearly, the risk is low.

Although clinical experience with intra-articular steroid therapy supports its safety, rapidly progressive joint failure has been observed after frequent, repeated injections in large doses into the same joint. The masking of pain by intra-articular steroid injections may lead to overuse, with subsequent breakdown and instability of the joint (analgesic arthropathy). Steroid injection may also damage articular cartilage directly. Weekly injections into rabbit joints resulted in degeneration of the articular cartilage, with fissures and cyst formation, associated with inhibition of the synthesis of

Figure 1 Improvement in pain score, as a percentage of baseline pain score, after intra-articular injection of glucocorticoid (a) or placebo (b). Combined results of several studies analyzed in Kirwan JR and Rankin E. Intra-articular therapy in osteoarthritis. *Baillière's Clin Rheumatol* 1997;11:769–94

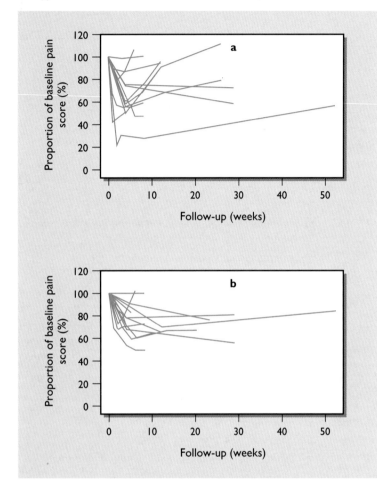

collagen and proteoglycans by the chondrocytes. Because of these concerns, intra-articular steroids are generally employed at intervals not shorter than 3–4 months.

Counterbalancing the possibility that excessive doses of intra-articular steroids and/or too frequent injection of steroid into the same joint may lead to joint damage, is the observation that intra-articular steroid injection ameliorates some of the pathologic changes of OA in animal models, raising the possibility that this therapy may be disease-modifying, in addition to any effect it may have on the palliation of joint pain. No evidence exists, however, that steroids favorably influence either the pathologic changes in articular cartilage or osteophytosis in humans with OA.

Some clinicians recommend weeks of joint rest (for example crutch walking) after an intra-articular steroid injection, while others permit the patient to return promptly to usual daily activities. The deleterious effects of intra-articular steroids on cartilage seen in a rabbit model of OA were potentiated by exercise, arguing in favor of a period of post-injection joint rest. Patients who were hospitalized and placed at rest after an intra-articular injection of steroids have been found to have had a longer duration of response than ambulatory patients. Many physicians caution the patient to minimize joint loading for a period of time following the

Figure 2 Triamcinolone hexacetonide crystals. (a) Rod-shaped unfragmented crystals with blunt, squared, or tapered ends and strong birefringence with negative elongation are indistinguishable from monosodium urate crystals. (b) Intracellular crystals of triamcinolone hexacetonide in synovial fluid obtained from a patient during a post-injection flare. Compensated polarized light x 400. From Schumacher HR, Reginato AJ. In *Atlas of Synovial Fluid Analysis and Crystal Identification*. Philadelphia: Lea & Febiger, 1991:1–257

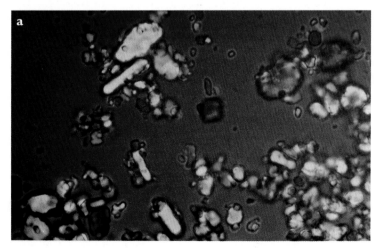

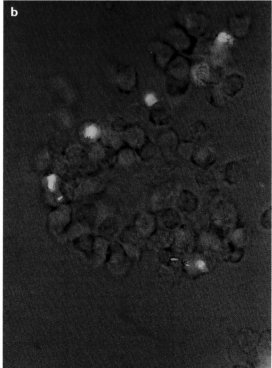

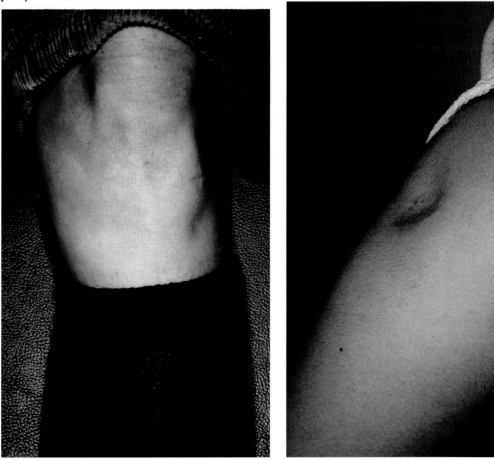

Figure 3 Cutaneous and subcutaneous atrophy after badly placed injection of a depot glucocorticoid preparation in a patient being treated for knee pain. Photograph courtesy of Jeffery Travers, MD

Figure 4 Cutaneous and subcutaneous atrophy after injection of a depot glucocorticoid preparation around the elbow. Photograph courtesy of Jeffery Travers, MD

Table 1 Placement of intra-articular steroid injections as revealed by concurrent injection of radiologic contrast medium

Joint	Extra-articular	Uncertain	Intra-articular
Knee	17	3	39
Shoulder	6	12	2
Wrist	2	2	4
Thumb carpometacarpal	1	2	0
Finger			
metacarpophalangeal	0	1	0
distal interphalangeal	0	1	0
Elbow	1	0	5
Ankle	3	0	6
Acromioclavicular	1	0	0
Total	**31**	**21**	**56**

Reproduced with permission from Jones A, Regan M, Ledingham J, et al. Importance of placement of intra-articular steroid injections. Br J Rheumatol 1993;307:1329–30

injection, even though controlled data to support this recommendation for patients are not available.

How important is accuracy in the placement of a joint injection? It would appear that injections are often inaccurate. In a study of patients receiving intra-articular steroid injections into a variety of joints, injections were shown by contrast radiography to be extra-articular in as many as 30% of cases (Table 1). Aspiration of joint fluid was associated with improved accuracy. Inaccuracy of the injection would not matter if it did not affect efficacy but, unfortunately, the same study suggested that inaccurate injections produced less improvement than those delivered into the joint space.

Which patient with OA is a candidate for intra-articular steroid injection? Several studies have failed to demonstrate any clear-cut predictors of response to corticosteroids other than, possibly, the presence of an effusion. (As indicated above, effusion may simply be a surrogate for the accuracy of the injection.) Although many authors suggest that intra-articular steroid injection in patients with OA should be reserved for those with acute synovitis, there are no data to support this view. It is reasonable to consider using a corticosteroid injection in patients who fail to respond to other conservative therapy and in those unwilling or unable to undergo surgery.

Finally, it should be recognized that OA pain may arise from para-articular structures. In those cases, injection of steroid into painful pericapsular sites and ligaments may produce symptomatic relief.

Bibliography

Gaffney K, Ledingham J, Perry JD. Intra-articular triamcinolone hexacetonide in knee osteoarthritis: factors influencing the clinical response. *Ann Rheum Dis* 1995;54:379–81

Jones A, Regan M, Ledingham J, *et al*. Importance of placement of intra-articular steroid injections. *Br Med J* 1993;307:1329–30

Neustadt DH. Intra-articular steroid therapy. In Moskowitz RW, Howell DS, Godberg VM, Mankin HF, eds. *Osteoarthritis: Diagnosis and Medical/Surgical Management.* Philadelphia: WB Saunders Co,1984:493–510

CHAPTER TWELVE

Local therapy for OA pain

III. Intra-articular injection of hyaluronic acid

Hyaluronan (HA) is a large, polydisperse linear glycosaminoglycan composed of repeating disaccharides of glucuronic acid and N-acetylglucosamine (Figure 1). Synoviocytes, fibroblasts and chondrocytes all synthesize HA, which is present in all mammalian connective tissues at concentrations of 0.05–5%, with an relative molecular mass (RMM) of 6×10^4–12×10^6 daltons (Da). Synovial fluid is a plasma ultrafiltrate modified by addition of a high concentration of HA, which is synthesized and secreted into the joint cavity by the type B cells of the synovial lining. In normal human synovial fluid the RMM of HA is 6–7×10^6 Da and the concentration 2–4 mg/ml.

In OA, the concentration and RMM of synovial fluid HA are reduced and the viscoelastic properties of the fluid compromised. Injection of exogenous HA into the joint presumably supplements the endogenous HA and has been reported to relieve joint pain in patients with OA, sometimes for many months (despite evidence that the injected HA is cleared from the joint in no more than a few days),

and to increase the RMM and quantity of HA synthesized by the synovium.

HA preparations marketed for intra-articular (IA) injection range from 0.25–2×10^6 Da and have been purified from rooster comb or human umbilical cord or have been produced by bacteria. To increase the average RMM, prolong its half-life within the joint and – it has been claimed – improve its clinical efficacy, HA has been modified to form hylans, chemically cross-linked HA molecules with an average RMM as high as 23×10^6 Da. One HA preparation, Hyalgan (RMM = 5–7.5×10^5 Da), and one hylan, Synvisc® (hylan G-F 20), have been approved by the Food and Drug Administration for use in humans with knee OA whose joint pain has not responded to nonmedicinal measures and analgesic drugs. Synvisc® is a highly purified formulation of rooster comb HA, the major portion of which is cross-linked with formaldehyde and the remainder with vinylsulfone to form a highly viscous gel, whose RMM is 6–7×10^6 Da. As indicated above, injected HA has a short residence time in the joint. For Hyalgan®, the half-life is 17 hours; the smaller component of Synvisc® (90% of the preparation) has a half-life of 1.5 days and the larger component, 8.8 days. Insufficient information is available to establish the optimal number of injections or the dose necessary for a successful therapeutic outcome or to permit direct comparison of the efficacy and adverse effects of the two HA preparations currently approved by the FDA for use in humans.

Possible mechanisms of action

HA molecules in solution form an extensive network. High RMM HA is viscoelastic, that is it behaves as a viscous liquid at low shear rates and an elastic

Figure 1 Chemical structure of hyaluronan. The molecule is a long-chain polymer consisting of repeating units of D-glucuronic acid and N-acetylglucosamine

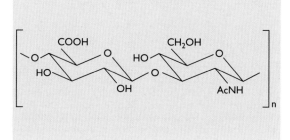

solid at high shear rates. Because of its HA content, joint fluid acts as a viscous lubricant during slow movement of the joint, as in walking, and as an elastic shock absorber during rapid movement, as in running. Various functions have been attributed to synovial fluid HA, including lubrication of the soft tissues (e.g. adjacent fronds of synovial villi) and formation of a surface layer on the articular cartilage. HA has a variety of effects on cells *in vitro* that may relate to its reported effects in joint disease. For example, it inhibits prostaglandin E-2 (PGE-2) synthesis induced by interleukin-1; protects against proteoglycan depletion and cytotoxicity induced by interleukin-1, mononuclear cell-conditioned medium and oxygen-derived free radicals; and affects leukocyte adherence, proliferation, migration and phagocytosis. Reduction of cellular damage by reactive oxygen species in the presence of HA has been attributed to two mechanisms: the first, competition between HA and cells for free radicals, is independent of the RMM of the HA while the second, prevention of contact between the target cell and enzymes that produce reactive oxygen, is proportional to the RMM of the HA. In addition, during degradation of HA by free radicals the latter are consumed in the reaction, reducing their concentration in the synovial fluid. HA has been shown to have a direct effect on control mechanisms of monocytes activation, for example it

increases mRNA expression for interleukin 1-β (IL-1β), tumor necrosis factor-α (TNF-α), and insulin-like growth factor-1 (IGF-1). Monoclonal antibodies against the HA receptor, CD44, block the effect of HA on the expression of IL-1β, TNF-α, and IGF-1, indicating a direct interaction of HA with the cell. In cartilage, HA has been shown to suppress extracellular matrix degradation by fibronectin fragments.

It is not clear whether any of the effects of HA on cultured cells are relevant to clinical outcomes after IA injection. Furthermore, it should be noted that the effects of exogenous HA on cellular activity *in vivo* are generally compared to activities in control cultures in which the medium contains little or no HA although, even in a diseased joint, the concentration of endogenous HA is 0.5–1 mg/ml and the average RMM 5×10^6 Da.

It has also been suggested that HA may modify fluid flow through the joint. A constant flow of HA occurs through the normal joint, with a half-life of 0.5 and 1.0 days in rabbits and sheep, respectively. Although it has been reported that the flow of synovial fluid is diminished in OA, most measurements indicate more rapid clearance of both HA and protein from inflamed joints, even when synovitis is mild, as in OA. Others have suggested that HA acts as a chemical sponge, binding or entangling both macromolecules and particulate debris in the diseased joint, and that the rapid clearance of

Table 1 Effects of intra-articular injection of Healon® on limiting viscosity and HA concentration of synovial fluid from human subjects

Sample	HA concentration, mg/ml		Limiting viscosity, cc/g	
	Mean ± SD	Range	Mean ± SD	Range
Healon®	10	10		2000–2500
Normal synovial fluid*	2.26 ± 0.13	1.45–2.94	5230 ± 140	4500–6000
OA synovial fluid				
pre-treatment	1.56 ± 0.36[a]	1.14–1.99[a]	3325 ± 650[b]	3000–4300[b]
post-treatment	1.73 ± 0.29[a]	1.38–2.14[a]	3825 ± 512[b]	3300–4500[b]
improvement with				
treatment	0.17 ± 0.27[a]	-0.39–0.42[a]	500 ± 316[b]	200–900[b]

*Values obtained on 71 joints from 42 donors, collected as 10 pooled samples and three individual samples. From Balazs EA, Watson D, Duff IF *et al.* Hyaluronic acid in synovial fluid. I. Molecular parameters of hyaluronic acid in normal and arthritis human fluids. *Arthr Rheum* 1967;10:357–76. [a]Values from seven patients enrolled in the study. From Peyron JG, Balasz EA. Preliminary clinical assessment of Na-hyaluronate injection into the human knee. *Pathol Biol* 1974;22:731–6; [b]values from four of the seven patients, in which intrinsic viscosity was measured 1 week after injection of Healon®

injected HA results in removal of these deleterious substances from the joint space. However, experimental manipulation of the RMM and concentration of HA in canine knee joints by injection of exogenous HA had no effect on the rate of clearance of radiolabelled albumin. There is little evidence that injection of HA promotes clearance of metabolites and debris or significantly augments the fluid flow through the joint. The original rationale proposed for IA HA treatment of OA was to increase the viscosity of the synovial fluid. It has been proposed that injection of an OA joint with HA or hylan restores the viscoelasticity of the synovial fluid, augments the flow of joint fluid, normalizes endogenous HA synthesis and/or inhibits HA degradation, and reduces joint pain. The investigators have contended that altered properties of synovial fluid contribute importantly to progression of joint destruction in OA and that transient supplementation of joint fluid leads to long-lasting increases in the RMM and concentration of endogenous HA, resulting in improved joint function. However, although the concept that viscosupplementation by IA injection of HA is useful in the treatment of OA is promoted by the manufacturers of the preparations currently marketed in the USA, few data exist to support this mechanism of action. Data from humans, in particular, are scarce. While the RMM of synovial fluid HA may increase temporarily after injection of exogenous HA, no evidence exists that this treatment returns either the concentration or the RMM of synovial fluid HA to a level approximating that in normal synovial fluid (Table 1) or, indeed, that any abnormality in synovial fluid HA leads to OA or progression of established joint damage.

Effects of HA injection on OA pain

Several investigations have concluded that IA injection of HA relieves joint pain and improves function in humans with knee OA. In 1997 Kirwan and Rankin reviewed published studies of the effects of IA HA therapy and compared outcomes with those obtained after IA injection of placebo or corticosteroid. The data indicate that joint aspiration alone improves knee pain in patients with OA. HA injections appear to result in improvement which is similar in magnitude to that of arthrocentesis or

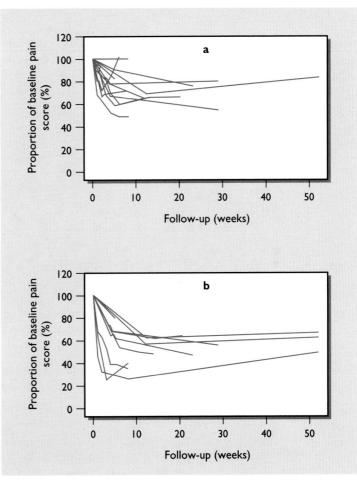

Figure 2 Improvement in pain score, relative to the baseline score, in several studies reviewed by Kirwan JR and Rankin E. (a) After intra-articular injection of placebo; (b) after intra-articular injection of hyaluronic acid. From Kirwan JR, Rankin E. Intra-articular therapy in osteoarthritis. *Baillière's Clin Rheumatol* 1997;11:769–94

placebo, but of somewhat greater duration. The magnitude of improvement after a series of IA HA injections appears to be comparable to that after an injection of steroid (Figure 2; compare with Figure 1 in intra-articular corticosteroid injection chapter). However, although the latter produces improvement more rapidly, the benefit appears to be more short-lived than after IA HA. Whether improvement after HA injection is due to a placebo effect or regression to the mean (i.e. selection of patients for IA injection whose symptoms are more severe than average, and whose pain would improve even without treatment) is unclear.

Considerable caution is required in interpreting the results of clinical trials of IA HA treatment.

Table 2 Level of pain, in mm, on a 100mm visual analog scale, after a 50-foot walk, results for all patients randomized

| Study group | Baseline | Study week | | | | | % Improvement in pain compared to baseline | | |
		12	16	26	Last observ'n		Week 12	Week 26	Last observ'n
HA, n	163	115	109	105	160		57	67	50
Mean (SD)	54(29)	23 (25)	21 (24)	18 (21)	27 (27)				
Placebo, n	167	129	123	113	163		56	56	49
Mean (SD)	55(29)	24 (26)	22 (25)	24 (27)	28 (30)				
Naproxen, n	162	125	119	111	160		61	61	54
Mean (SD)	54(28)	21 (25)	24 (28)	21 (25)	25 (28)				

Modified from Altman RD, Moskowitz R and the Hyalgan Study Group. Intra-articular sodium hyaluronate (Hyalgan) in the treatment of patients with osteoarthritis of the knee: a randomized clinical trial. J Rheumatol 1998;25:2203–12

In particular, the magnitude and duration of the placebo response to IA injections is large and may be sustained for 6 months or longer (Figure 2), making evaluation of any IA therapy difficult. It is not clear that the difference between HA and placebo, even if statistically significant, is clinically significant.

By way of illustration, a recently reported study in which patients were treated with 5 weekly IA injections of HA or saline or with naproxen, 500 mg/bid, serves to emphasize the vigor of the placebo response to IA injections. Subjects who received IA injections were given dummy tablets, as a control for the naproxen, while subjects in the naproxen arm received 5 weekly subcutaneous injections of lidocaine, as a blind for the IA injections. Among patients who completed the study (approximately 67%), a decrease in knee pain after a 50-feet walk of 20 mm [on a 100 mm visual analog scale (VAS)] was seen in 56% of those who received HA and 41% of the placebo group. Twenty-six weeks after initiation of treatment, 47.6% of patients in the HA group but only 33.1% of those in the saline group were pain-free or reported only mild pain (p = 0.039). Results in the HA group were similar to those in the naproxen group. The authors concluded that treatment with HA was as effective as naproxen for patients with knee OA and had fewer side-effects.

However, an intention-to-treat analysis of all subjects randomized to treatment (rather than of only the completers) showed that the series of IA saline injections was as effective as the positive control, naproxen (Table 2). The failure to demonstrate superiority of naproxen over placebo in this study stands in sharp contrast to the results of virtually every published placebo-controlled trial of an NSAID, in which the NSAID produces greater relief of OA pain than placebo. However, a distinction must be made: in the typical NSAID study the placebo is a dummy tablet or capsule which mirrors the active NSAID in color, size, shape and odor; in studies of HA the placebo is a series of IA injections of saline or the vehicle.

Furthermore, the large placebo response is by no means the only important limitation of the clinical trials which have reported a positive effect of IA HA therapy. For example, in some studies the person who performed the patient evaluations was not blinded with respect to the treatment group, raising the possibility that bias was introduced because the HA and saline control solutions are so readily distinguished from each other by the marked differences in their viscosity.

In a study in which the authors concluded that HA treatment was superior to placebo, a decrease in synovial effusion was the major outcome measure. However, the severity of joint pain and mean volume of synovial effusion at baseline were both significantly greater in the HA group than in the placebo group and synovial effusion volumes in both treatment groups were substantial (18.5 ± 14.0 cc vs, 13.9 ± 9.6 cc) – much larger than is characteristic of OA. Synovial fluid analyses were not reported, but these relatively large effusion volumes raise the possibility that, at least in some cases, the arthropathy was due to some cause other than OA (e.g. gout, calcium pyrophosphate dihydrate crystal deposition disease). Furthermore, effusion volume has not been validated as an outcome measure in OA clinical trials; because of the difficulty in completely aspirating a knee effusion it is not well suited for this purpose.

Although the above discussion emphasizes the large placebo response in clinical trials of IA HA, it should be noted that several preclinical studies suggest an analgesic effect which cannot readily be attributed to a placebo response, although they provide no insight into possible underlying mechanisms. However, relief of joint pain for months after the injected material has been cleared from the joint, as has been reported in some clinical trials in humans, is difficult to explain by any mechanism, whether it be biochemical, physicochemical, or mechanical.

Disease-modifying effects of IA HA injection

Preclinical data are contradictory with respect to whether IA injection of HA modifies the progression of joint damage in OA and, if so, whether treatment is beneficial or detrimental. Numerous relevant methodological differences exist among the animal studies which have examined this issue: in addition to the species used, the duration of treatment, source and RMM of the HA, timing of the intervention (prophylactic or therapeutic) and the outcome measures employed may all influence the results. Furthermore, as discussed below, one study in a canine model of OA and another in an ovine model raise a concern that, rather than protecting against joint damage in OA, HA injection into the joint may, in fact, accelerate joint degeneration.

When dogs which had undergone anterior cruciate ligament transection (ACLT) were treated prophylactically with a series of IA injections of HA, no effect on morphologic changes of OA was apparent. However, a striking reduction in the proteoglycan concentration of the articular cartilage (as reflected by the cartilage uronic acid concentration) was seen in every dog 7 weeks after the last HA injection (Table 3). Although mechanical testing of the cartilage was not performed in the above study, because the stiffness of articular cartilage is directly proportional to its PG concentration this finding raises a concern that HA treatment could accelerate joint damage in OA.

In support of this possibility, IA injection of HA in sheep which had undergone meniscectomy resulted in significantly more extensive osteophytosis and cartilage fibrillation, and a reduction in the net rate of PG synthesis by the OA cartilage, in comparison with OA joints of sheep which had been injected with saline. As indicated above, forceplate data indicate that the increase in severity of joint pathology after injection of the canine OA knee with HA was associated with an increase in loading of the arthritic knee, consistent with 'analgesic

Table 3 Compositional analysis of femoral condylar cartilage from the osteoarthritic knee of dogs which had undergone ACLT

Treatment group	Source of cartilage	Water content		Uronic acid concentration	
		% Dry weight	OA knee: contra knee	µg/mg dry weight	OA knee: contra knee
IA Saline injection (n = 6)	Medial condyle	73.3 ± 3.1	1.05 ± 0.05	5.5 ± 1.0	1.4 ± 0.4
	Lateral condyle	76.2 ± 2.7	1.07 ± 0.04	5.6 ± 0.8	1.3 ± 0.2
	Medial trochlea	78.5 ± 1.8	1.12 ± 0.07	3.2 ± 0.8	1.6 ± 0.5
IA HA injection (n = 6)	Medial condyle	72.9 ± 1.5	1.05 ± 0.04	3.9 ± 1.1	0.8 ± 0.2
	Lateral condyle	74.7 ± 2.4	1.02 ± 0.07	3.2 ± 1.6	0.7 ± 0.3
	Medial trochlea	77.3 ± 0.9	1.11 ± 0.03	2.2 ± 0.9	0.9 ± 0.4

Contra, contralateral; IA, intra-articular; HA, hyaluronan. From Smith G Jr, Myers SI, Brandt KD, Mickler EA. Effect of intra-articular hyaluronan injection in experimental canine osteoarthritis. *Arthritis Rheum* 1998;41:976–85

arthropathy[1]. Hurwitz *et al.* have reported that the adductor moment at the knee in patients with medial compartment knee OA was greater while they were taking an NSAID than after withdrawal from the drug, when their knee pain was more severe, i.e. pharmacologic amelioration of joint pain resulted in an increase in mechanical loading of the damaged joint.

Insufficient information is available to permit a conclusion concerning the effect of this treatment, if any, on the progression of OA in humans. In the single clinical trial which has examined this question, 36 patients with knee OA were treated conventionally or with weekly injections of Hyalgan® for 3 consecutive weeks every 3 months (a total of 12 injections). Based upon arthroscopic observations at baseline and again one year later, Listrat *et al.* concluded that HA treatment slowed the progression of chondropathy. However, that conclusion must be tempered by the relatively small number of patients in the study, the fact that the HA group exhibited less severe chondropathy at baseline than those treated conventionally, and the fact that the proportion of patients who required an NSAID during the study was twice as great in the control as in the HA group. Furthermore, although arthroscopy is useful for the observation of damage to menisci, ligaments and the articular surface, it is not a good tool with which to detect anatomic or biochemical changes in the OA joint and it cannot be considered to have an accurate, sensitive, reproducible and validated outcome measure for evaluation of chondropathy in OA. Cartilage thickness and the mechanical quality of the cartilage cannot be assessed unless a striking loss of cartilage has occurred. Probing the cartilage can provide some information about the resilience of the tissue, but the probe assesses change in only a small area and cannot simulate the effects of load bearing.

Safety

Is IA HA therapy safe? Certainly, it carries none of the concerns associated with systemic inhibition of prostaglandin synthesis by NSAIDs. Local reactions at the injection site, with pain, tenderness and erythema, are generally transient and require little more than reassurance of the patient and an ice pack. However, some reports have suggested a relatively high incidence of local reactions following treatment with hylan G-F 20. In a study of 22 patients who received a total of 88 injections into 28 knees, post-injection flares occurred in 27% of patients and after 11% of injections. In some cases acute synovitis was associated with joint swelling lasting up to 3 weeks and the synovial fluid leukocyte count exceeded 50 000 cells per mm^3, raising concern about the presence of acute bacterial infection, although bacterial cultures of the synovial fluid and crystal analysis were negative (Table 4). In a few cases, however, IA injection of HA has been followed promptly by an acute attack of pseudogout, confirmed by the identification of weakly positively birefringent crystals in the synovial fluid. No direct comparisons are available of the incidence of local reactions after IA injection of hylan G-F 20

Table 4 Analysis of synovial fluid from patients experiencing an acute local reaction after intra-articular injection of hylan G-F 20

Patient number	Injection number	Days after injection	Volume aspirated ml	Synovial fluid leukocyte count/mm^3	% Polymorphonuclear leukocytes
1	4	5	10	13 000	52
2	4	6	10	5000	44
3	5	2	40	20 700	26
4	3	13	8	6200	34
	3	13	8	6200	34
	5	2	30	38 000	61
	6	1	NR	75 000	84

Crystal examination and bacterial cultures were negative in each case; NR, not recorded. Adapted from Puttick MPE, Wade JP, Chalmers A, *et al.* Acute local reactions after intra-articular hylan for osteoarthritis of the knee. *J Rheumatol* 1995;22:1311–14 and that after injection of other HA preparations, arthrocentesis alone, or corticosteroid.

Although, in the short run, IA HA therapy seems safe (except, perhaps, for the occasional 'pseudoseptic' reaction as indicated above) force-plate studies in animals suggest that overloading of the damaged joint may occur after this treatment which may lead to depletion of PGs in articular cartilage and could, in the long run, increase structural damage of the joint. Given the increasing use of HA in humans, this is an important area for further study.

Bibliography

Altman RD, Moskowitz R and the Hyalgan Study Group. Intra-articular sodium hyaluronate (Hyalgan) in the treatment of patients with osteoarthritis of the knee: a randomized clinical trial. *J Rheumatol* 1998;25:2203–12

Balazs EA, Denlinger JL. Viscosupplementation: a new concept in the treatment of osteoarthritis. *J Rheumatol* 1993;20(suppl 39):3–9

Brandt KD, Smith GN, Simon LS. A review: intra-articular injection of hyaluronic acid as treatment for knee osteoarthritis. What is the evidence? *Arthritis Rheum* 2000;43:1192–1203

Ghosh P, Read R, Armstrong S, *et al.* The effects of intraarticular administration of hyaluronan in a model of early osteoarthritis in sheep. I. Gait analysis and radiological and morphological studies. *Semin Arthritis Rheum* 1993;22(6 Suppl 1):18–30

Ghosh P, Read R, Numata Y, *et al.* The effects of intraarticular administration of hyaluronan in a model of early osteoarthritis in sheep. II. Cartilage composition and proteoglycan metabolism. *Semin Arthritis Rheum* 1993;22(6 Suppl 1):31–42

Hurwitz DE, Sharma L, Andriacchi TP. Effect of knee pain on joint loading in patients with osteoarthritis. *Curr Opin Rheumatol* 1999;11:422–6

Jones AC, Pattricj M, Doherty S, Doherty M. Intra-articular hyaluronic acid compared to intra-articular triamcinolone hexacetonide in inflammatory knee osteoarthritis. *Osteoarthritis Cartilage* 1995;3:269–73

Kirwan JR, Rankin E. Intra-articular therapy in osteoarthritis. *Baillière's Clin Rheumatol* 1997;11:769–94

Listrat V, Ayral X, Patarnello F, *et al.* Arthroscopic evaluation of potential structure modifying activity of hyaluronan (Hyalgan) in osteoarthritis of the knee. *Osteoarthritis Cartilage* 1997;5:153–60

Puttick MPE, Wade JP, Chalmers A, *et al.* Acute local reactions after intra-articular hylan for osteoarthritis of the knee. *J Rheumatol* 1995;22:1311–14

Smith GN Jr, Myers SL, Brandt KD, Mickler EA. Effect of IA hyaluronan injection in experimental canine osteoarthritis. *Arthritis Rheum* 1998;41:976–85

CHAPTER THIRTEEN

A rational strategy for selecting the initial pharmacologic agent for the management of osteoarthritis pain

The evidence supports the recommendation that acetaminophen (ACET) should be prescribed initially, in a dose up to 4000 mg/d, in parallel with implementation of nonpharmacologic measures appropriate for the individual patient. Although some contend that the presence of clinical signs of inflammation (e.g. warmth or erythema over the joint, synovial effusion) warrants initial treatment with an NSAID, rather than an analgesic, there is no evidence to support that view. ACET may be as effective as an NSAID in osteoarthritis (OA) patients with clinical signs of joint inflammation (e.g. joint swelling and tenderness) or histologic evidence of synovitis as in those in whom these are absent.

Given their potential adverse effects and cost (Table 1), and the fact that no drug has been shown to prevent, delay progression of, or reverse the pathologic changes of OA in humans, drugs should serve an adjunctive or complementary, rather than primary, role in the management of OA pain. Nonpharmacologic measures (Table 2) are as important as – and often more important than – drug treatment. A health education program designed to assist patients with self-management can reduce pain and decrease health care costs. Furthermore, the benefits may persist for years.

It is clear that some patients experience greater relief of knee pain with an NSAID than with ACET. However, there is no way to predict which OA patient will obtain greater benefit from an NSAID than from an analgesic. The evidence suggests that ACET is at least as effective as an NSAID in relieving joint pain in nearly 50% of patients with OA. In a survey of 668 patients with OA of the hip or knee

Table 1 Approximate retail cost, in US dollars, for 30 days of treatment of osteoarthritis pain with various regimens

	Pharmacy A	Pharmacy B	Pharmacy C	Pharmacy D
Acetaminophen, generic, 3 g/d				
tablets	11.14	7.18	8.98	8.98
caplets	11.14	7.18	8.98	8.98
gel caps	11.86	7.18	10.60	10.78
Celecoxib, 200 mg/d	73.04	62.99	84.00	72.99
Rofecoxib, 12.5 mg/d	73.13	70.20	84.00	74.55
Rofecoxib, 25 mg/d	73.14	70.20	84.00	74.55
Naproxen, generic, 750 mg/d	20.39	16.59	26.29	17.90
Naproxen, generic, 1000 mg/d	20.69	19.99	30.59	23.99
Naproxen, generic, 1000 mg/d + misoprostol, 800 μg/d	138.78	135.96	72.58	146.38
Naproxen, generic, 1000 mg/d + omeprazole, 20 mg/d	141.98	123.28	155.58	139.98

Retail cost in four Indianapolis pharmacies in January 2000

who were asked to compare the effectiveness of, and their overall satisfaction with, ACET, relative to NSAIDs which they had received, approximately 45% reported that ACET was about as effective as, or more effective than, their NSAID. A comparable proportion of patients reported that they were as satisfied, or more satisfied, with ACET as with the NSAIDs which they had received (Table 3).

The use of ACET in a dose up to 4000 mg/d as the initial drug of choice for the systemic treatment of OA pain is consistent with the 1995 American College of Rheumatology Guidelines for Management of OA, which state: "Toxicity is the major reason for not recommending the use of NSAIDs as first-line therapy for patients with OA". The serious adverse events associated with NSAIDs (especially those related to inhibition of COX-1, such as gastric or duodenal ulcers, gastrointestinal bleeding, renal insufficiency, inhibition of platelet aggregation) are not seen with ACET.

It is possible that large-scale clinical trials currently in progress will show that the striking reduction in the incidence of gastroduodenal ulceration after administration of specific COX-2 inhibitors will be accompanied by a corresponding decrease in clinically important adverse GI events, such as bleeding, ulceration and perforation. However, even if that proves to be the case, nonselective NSAIDs and specific COX-2 inhibitors are associated with other adverse effects, such as renal insufficiency, edema and congestive heart failure. Furthermore, the incidence of nonspecific GI side-effects (e.g. dsypepsia, abdominal pain) with specific COX-2 inhibitors may not be appreciably different from that seen with nonselective NSAIDs.

Table 2 Nonpharmacologic measures for the management of osteoarthritis pain

Instruction of the patient in principles of joint protection

Thermal modalities

Isometric exercises to strengthen periarticular muscles in patients with knee OA

Weight reduction, if the patient is obese

Avoidance of excessive loading of the arthritic hip or knee by use of a cane or walker

Shoes with well-cushioned soles

Orthotics for the patient with varus or valgus knee deformity

Medial taping of the patella for patients with patellofemoral OA

The safety profiles of the new specific COX-2 inhibitors are less favorable than that of ACET and they are much more expensive than ACET (Table 1). Hence they should not be considered alternatives to ACET as a first-line drug for OA pain. However, if sufficient improvement in symptoms does not result within a reasonable time (e.g. 4 weeks) after initiation of treatment with ACET and implementation of appropriate nonpharmacologic measures, a low dose of NSAID may be added. If risk factors for serious adverse GI side-effects of NSAIDs are present and a nonselective NSAID is used – even in low dose – it is reasonable to co-administer a gastroprotective agent, such as misoprostol or a proton pump inhibitor. As an alternative, tramadol or a weak opioid may be considered. If this does not produce sufficient symptomatic relief, nonmedicinal measures should be continued and an NSAID prescribed

Table 3 Effectiveness of acetaminophen, compared to NSAID, and overall satisfaction (effectiveness and side-effects) with acetaminophen versus NSAIDs reported by patients with hip or knee OA: per cent of patients in each category

Patients' judgement	Much less	Somewhat less	About the same	More	Much More	Total
Effectiveness	33	23	30	12	3	101
Satisfaction	32	20	32	13	3	100

From Wolfe F, Zhao S, Lane N. Preference for nonsteroidal antiinflammatory drugs over acetaminophen by rheumatic disease patients: a survey of 1799 patients with osteoarthritis, rheumatoid arthritis, and fibromyalgia. *Arthritis Rheum* 2000;43:378–85

Figure 1 Algorithm for symptomatic treatment of patient with knee osteoarthritis. TF, tibiofemoral; PF, patellofemoral

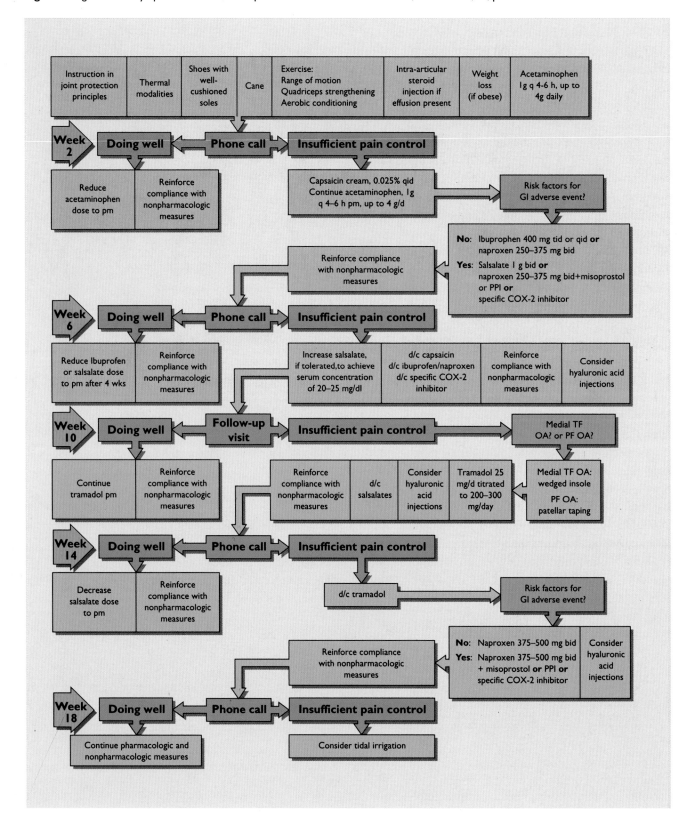

in an anti-inflammatory dose. Although specific COX-2 inhibitors are no more effective in relieving OA pain than nonselective NSAIDs in patients at high risk for an NSAID-associated GI catastrophe, a COX-2-specific NSAID may be preferable to even a low dose of a nonselective COX inhibitor.

As an alternative to the above strategy, a nonacetylated salicylate (e.g. salsalate, choline magnesium trisalicylate) may be prescribed. Because these drugs have minimal effects on systemic prostaglandin synthesis they do not cause the renal toxicity or inhibition of platelet aggregation associated with other NSAIDs. Furthermore, the incidence of serious GI side-effects with nonacetylated salicylates is lower than that with nonselective COX-2 inhibitors, while they are as effective as the latter in relieving OA pain. However, ototoxicity and central nervous system toxicity may limit the utility of salicylates in the older patient.

Because the risk of an NSAID-associated GI catastrophe is dose-dependent, when nonselective NSAIDs are used the lowest effective dose should be employed. Increases in dose are not necessarily accompanied by increases in efficacy. In general, higher doses should be avoided in most patients with OA. The analgesia produced by ACET and that achieved with an NSAID may be additive, so that concomitant use of ACET may permit a reduction in the daily dose of NSAID.

Figure 1 depicts an algorithmic approach to the treatment of a newly diagnosed patient with knee OA. The progressive levels of treatment are associated with increasing cost, decreasing convenience for the patient, and an increasing risk of side-effects. It should be emphasized that the scheme should not be followed dogmatically. Treatment must be individualized and flexibility is essential. The patient and physician should understand that for most patients with OA the goals of decreasing joint pain, increasing mobility and achieving a better quality of life are realistic and attainable.

CHAPTER FOURTEEN

Disease-modifying drugs for osteoarthritis (DMOADs)

As already discussed, for many patients with osteoarthritis (OA) symptomatic treatment with a nonsteroidal anti-inflammatory drug (NSAID) or analgesic may achieve some reduction in joint pain but, because of limitations in efficacy, cost and/or side-effects, is by no means satisfactory. Interest has arisen, therefore, in the possibility of pharmacologically modifying the disease process. Drugs that may prevent or retard progression of OA are now receiving increasing attention. A number of pharmacologic agents have been shown to reduce proteolytic breakdown of articular cartilage and/or to stimulate

matrix repair in animal models of OA in which morphologic, biochemical and metabolic changes in the OA cartilage mimic, more or less closely, those in human OA cartilage. Such agents have been called 'chondroprotective' drugs. However, because not only the cartilage, but all of the tissues of the joint are involved in this disease, it has been suggested recently that a preferable label is disease-modifying OA drug (DMOAD) (Figure 1).

DMOADs range from empirical compounds, for example tissue extracts, to site-specific metalloproteinase inhibitors designed by structural

Figure 1 It is anticipated that administration of a disease-modifying osteoarthritis drug (DMOAD) at a relatively early stage of structural damage, e.g. as in the radiograph depicted in (a), will retard or prevent progression to an advanced stage of joint damage, e.g. as seen in (b), which depicts marked loss of articular cartilage and bony sclerosis

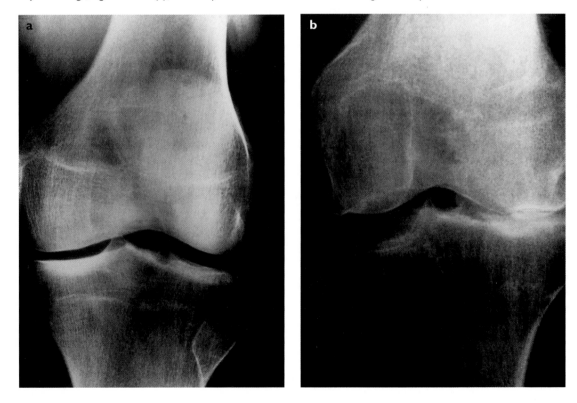

analysis to fit precisely into the catalytic site of the enzyme. Some of the agents reported to exhibit a DMOAD effect are tribenoside, tamoxifen, diacerhein, chloroquine, hyaluronic acid, glucocorticoids, tranexamic acid, heparinoids (e.g. glycosaminoglycan polysulfate [GAGPS], pentosan polysulfate [PPS], glycosaminoglycan peptide-complex [GP-C]), NSAIDs and doxycycline. Several of the agents receiving current attention are discussed below.

Nonsteroidal anti-inflammatory drugs

Claims that NSAIDs have DMOAD activity are based almost exclusively on *in vitro* evidence that the drug may modify proteoglycan or collagen metabolism, cytokine-mediated matrix degeneration, release or activity of matrix metalloproteinases (MMPs), and/or the actions of toxic oxygen metabolites. The number of *in vivo* studies of NSAIDs in experimental models of OA is remarkably limited, because all of the animal species which are commonly employed as models (e.g. the dog, the mouse, the rabbit, the guinea pig) are markedly sensitive to the gastrointestinal side-effects of NSAIDs and develop gastrointestinal hemorrhage or perforation before the joint pathology is well established.

On the other hand, some NSAIDs inhibit the synthesis of proteoglycans by chondrocytes *in vitro* and some, such as salicylate, rather than exhibiting a protective effect, have been shown to accelerate the progression of cartilage degeneration *in vivo* in animal models of OA. In humans, *in vivo* evidence that NSAIDs exhibit DMOAD activity is no less adequate than that in animal models.

It has also been contended that indomethacin, rather than exhibiting a DMOAD effect, may, in fact, accelerate joint damage in patients with knee OA. An increase in the rate of joint-space narrowing (implying loss of articular cartilage) has been reported in radiographs of patients with hip OA who were treated with that drug in comparison with those who received the weak COX inhibitor, azapropazone, and patients in the indomethacin group came to arthroplasty sooner than those in the azapropazone group. However, that study had several limitations: baseline pain scores were higher in the azapropazone group than in the indomethacin group, and the timing of joint replacement surgery was not based on well-defined clinical criteria but

was determined by a physician who was not blinded to the treatment group. Furthermore, even though the azapropazone group had higher post-treatment pain scores, they were deemed to be surgical candidates later in their course of treatment than the indomethacin group, suggesting a bias to delay surgery.

In support of the contention that indomethacin is detrimental in OA, results of a clinical trial in humans led to the conclusion that this NSAID accelerated joint breakdown in patients with knee OA. In a double-blind, parallel study in which 376 patients with knee OA completed at least 1 year of treatment with indomethacin, 75 mg/d, tiaprofenic acid, 600 mg/d, or placebo, more than twice as many patients in the indomethacin group showed narrowing of the joint space in serial radiographs of the OA knee as those in the placebo group. However, a number of concerns exist relative to the design of that study. In summary, while the conclusion that indomethacin use leads to an acceleration of joint breakdown in patients with OA may be correct, the supporting evidence is not wholly convincing.

Heparinoids

Glycosaminoglycan polysulfate (Arteparon®) – an aqueous extract of bovine tracheal and bronchial cartilages which contains synthetically oversulfated chondroitin-4-sulfate and chondroitin-6-sulfate and 3 mg/ml of peptides – stimulates cartilage matrix synthesis and is a pan-protease inhibitor. Glycosaminoglycan peptide-complex (Rumalon®), an aqueous extract of calf cartilage and bone marrow, when constituted in solution contains approximately 1.8 mg/ml glycosaminoglycans, which are principally chondroitin-4-sulfate and chondroitin-6-sulfate and 0.7 mg/ml peptide. *In vivo* studies in animal models of OA have shown a DMOAD effect with both of these agents.

Several clinical trials have reported the efficacy of GAGPS in patients with OA. For example, in a study of the effects of GAGPS in patients with OA who also received NSAIDs, outcomes were compared to those in patients treated with NSAIDs alone or with GP-C plus NSAIDs. Although X-ray progression of OA was reported to be slower in both active treatment groups than in the controls, failure to include a placebo group or to control for

Figure 2 Evidence of the protective effect of doxycycline when administered orally in a canine cruciate deficiency model of OA. In the untreated dogs (a), articular cartilage on the distal femoral condyle of the unstable knee showed extensive full-thickness ulceration; cartilage from the same area of dogs (b) which received doxycycline was, in some cases, grossly normal, as seen in this figure; in other cases, it showed only slight pitting or thinning; scale in cm. From Yu LP Jr, Smith GN Jr, Brandt KD, *et al.* Reduction of the severity of canine osteoarthritis by prophylactic treatment with oral doxycycline. *Arthritis Rheum* 1992;35:1150–9

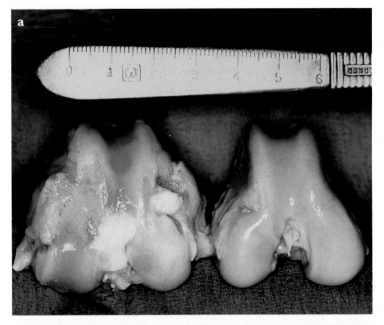

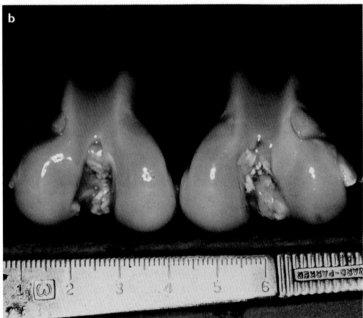

NSAID use cast serious doubt on the significance of the findings. A recent study, however, failed to confirm that GP-C has a DMOAD effect in patients with knee OA.

The fact that GAGPS and GP-C are derived from bovine tissues raised some concerns over the possible transmission of bovine spongiform encephalopathy. In addition, their lack of efficacy as DMOADs in adequately controlled human trials, bleeding complications related to the heparinoid structure of GAGPS, and cases of anaphylaxis related to the presence of antigenic protein components has resulted in removal of both of these agents from clinical use.

In contrast to GAGPS and GP-C, the heparinoid sodium pentosan polysulfate (PPS, SP54), a polysaccharide sulfate ester prepared from beech hemicellulose, lacks antigenic protein constituents. PPS has a mean relative molecular mass of 6000 Da and is a potent inhibitor of MMPs, leukocyte elastase and hyaluronidase. Several studies have shown that treatment with PPS can preserve the proteoglycan concentration of articular cartilage and help maintain cartilage integrity in various animal models of OA.

Calcium PPS, which has the advantage of being well absorbed after oral administration, has been shown to reduce loss of cartilage proteoglycans in animal models. In humans with OA of the finger joints it produced significant symptomatic relief in comparison with placebo. It remains to be demonstrated, however, that pentosans have a DMOAD effect in humans.

Tetracyclines

Based on prior observations that activities of MMPs (e.g. collagenase, gelatinase or stromelysin) are increased in OA articular cartilage and studies showing that tetracyclines inhibit MMPs, researchers have examined the effects of doxycycline on MMP activity *in vitro* and shown that doxycycline inhibited the activities of both gelatinase and collagenase in a concentration-dependent fashion.

This observation led to studies in a canine model of OA which showed that cartilage ulcerations on the medial femoral condyles could be prevented by prophylactic daily oral administration of doxycycline, 3.5 mg/kg (Figure 2). In other dogs, only mild pitting of the articular cartilage or some partial thinning was observed. Reductions in levels of both total and active collagenase and total and active gelatinase in extracts of cartilage from the OA knee were seen in samples from the active treatment group (Figure 3). Even when treatment was delayed until 4 weeks after cruciate ligament transection, a protective effect was seen.

Studies of the mechanism(s) by which doxycycline inhibits MMP activity have suggested that it alters the conformation of procollagenase, rendering it more susceptible to breakdown in the tissue. In addition, tetracyclines may interact with the zinc atom located at the catalytic site in MMPs or with the calcium atoms which provide conformational stability to the enzyme, resulting, in the latter case, in fragmentation of the proenzyme. This effect accounts for the observation that treatment with doxycycline led to reductions not only in the levels of active MMPs (e.g. gelatinase and collagenase) in extracts of OA cartilage, but also in the levels of total gelatinase and collagenase (Figure 4). However, doxycycline is not a particularly potent inhibitor of any of the MMPs that appear to be involved in cartilage destruction in OA and is unlikely to inhibit these enzymes *in vivo* at the tissue concentrations achieved after oral administration. More probably, the remarkable protective effect which this drug demonstrates in animal models of OA involves control of the expression of MMPs through inhibition of transcription or inhibition of translation.

Recent studies suggest yet another possible mechanism by which doxycycline may protect against cartilage breakdown involving nitric oxide (NO). It has been shown that NO is released spontaneously from OA cartilage in quantities large enough to cause tissue damage. A number of potentially detrimental effects of NO on articular cartilage have been elucidated: for example, NO may modulate the effects of interleukin-1 (IL-1) on cartilage matrix turnover. It suppresses extracellular matrix synthesis and has been implicated in the regulation of MMP production and activation of the latent proenzymes. In addition, it inhibits chrondrocyte proliferation and induces chrondrocyte death (Table 1). It has recently been shown that tetracyclines block the RNA expression and translation of the enzyme nitric oxide synthase (NOS),

Figure 3 Reductions in levels of total and active gelatinase in extracts of OA cartilage from dogs which had been treated with doxycycline, 3.5 mg/kg daily

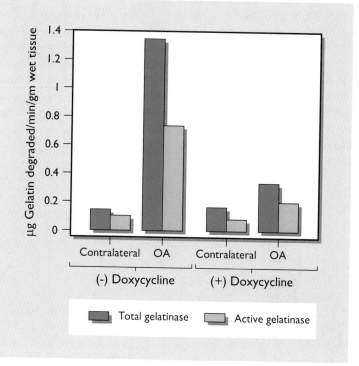

Figure 4 Effects of doxycycline on activation of neutrophil collagenase by trypsin. Lane 1 shows a prominent 55 kDa band, reflecting the latent proenzyme. Lane 2 shows the presence of a prominent 46 kDa band, reflecting active collagenase, produced by incubation of the latent enzyme with trypsin. Lane 3 shows the generation of several smaller, enzymatically inactive, fragments of the enzyme, which were generated when the proenzyme was activated with trypsin in the presence of doxycycline, 30 μg/ml

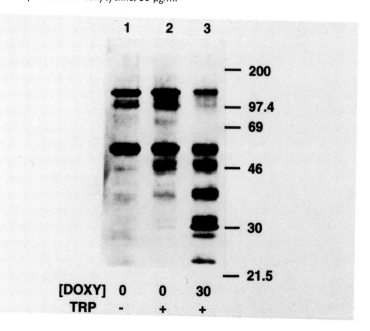

Table I Nitric oxide effects on chondrocyte proliferation and survival

Inhibition of collagen synthesis

Inhibition of proteoglycan synthesis

Inhibition of production of IL-1 receptor antagonist

Interference with integrin signaling

Induction of chondrocyte apoptosis

Stimulation of production and activation of matrix metalloproteinases

Inactivation of tissue inhibitors of matrix metalloproteinases (TIMPs)

Reproduced with permission from Lotz M. The role of nitric oxide in articular cartilage damage. In Brandt KD, ed. *Rheum Dis Clin North Am* Philadelphia, PA: WB Saunders, 1999:269–82

although they have no significant effect on NOS activity (Figure 5). Thus, tetracyclines may protect articular cartilage from enzymatic degradation both by direct effects on MMPs and by a more proximal effect, that is preventing the synthesis of NOS. In support of this possibility, treatment with N-imi-noethyl-L-lysine (L-NIL), a selective inhibitor of inducible NOS, reduced the severity of cartilage damage, synovial inflammation and osteophytosis, and the activities of collagenase and other metallo-proteinases in cartilage and synovial fluid in a canine model of OA.

Reports that the severity of cartilage damage in guinea pig and rabbit models of OA was reduced by oral administration of tetracycline support the above observations in the canine model of OA. These encouraging results have led to the implementation of a placebo-controlled multicenter clinical trial in humans to ascertain whether treatment with doxy-cycline can prevent the development of joint damage OA in knees at high risk for incident OA and/or slow the progression of OA in joints in which damage is already present.

Figure 5 Inhibition by doxycycline and minocycline of mRNA for inducible nitric oxide synthase (iNOS) by cells stimulated with lipopolysaccharide (LPS). mRNA for cyclo-oxygenase-2 (COX-2) was uninhibited under identical conditions, while hydrocortisone inhibited generation of the message for both iNOS and COX-2. Reproduced with permission from Amin AR, Attur MG, Thakker GD, *et al.* A novel mechanism of action of tetracyclines: effects on nitric oxide synthases. *Proc Natl Acad Sci USA* 1996;93:14014–18; ©1996, National Academy of Sciences, USA

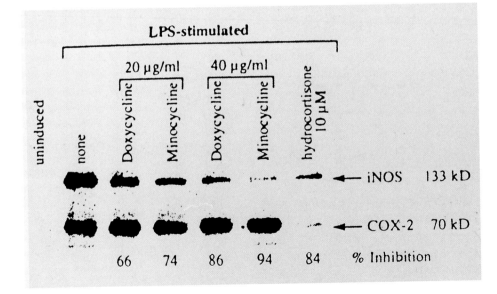

Diacerhein

Diacerhein, which is derived from rhubarb, is the acetylated form of the anthraquinone rhein. It has been shown to inhibit the expression of collagenase by chondrocytes exposed to interleukin-1 and to stimulate synthesis of prostaglandin E_2 by chondrocytes in culture, but has no effect on phospholipase A_2, cyclo-oxygenase or 5-lipoxygenase. Diacerhein has been reported to be effective in palliating symptoms of OA in humans, although beneficial effects are usually not seen with treatment periods shorter than 1 month. In the canine-cruciate deficiency model of OA, chondropathy in the unstable knee, as assessed arthroscopically 16 weeks after transection of the anterior cruciate ligament and by direct observation 32 weeks after surgery, was significantly less severe in the diacerhein treatment group (Figure 6).

In a recent 3-year placebo-controlled trial of diacerhein in humans with hip OA in which the dropout rate, unfortunately, was approximately

Table 2 Association* between radiographic progression of knee osteoarthritis (medial tibiofemoral compartment) and changes in overall knee pain over 3 years

Radiographic feature	Radiographic Progression	Joint pain	
		Worse	Better
Joint space narrowing	Yes	1	7
	No	15	41
			$p = 0.677$
Osteophytosis	Yes	1	7
	No	11	33
			$p = 0.663$
Sclerosis	Yes	0	3
	No	15	42
			$p = 0.566$

*Fisher's exact test. From Dieppe PA, Cushnaghan J, Shepstone L. The Bristol 'OA 500' study: progression of osteoarthritis (OA) over 3 years and the relationship between clinical and radiographic changes in the knee joint. *Osteoarthritis Cartilage* 1997:5:87–97

Figure 6 Progression of osteoarthritis from week 16 to week 32 after anterior cruciate ligament transection. Each dog was examined arthroscopically at 16 weeks, at which time an SFA (Société Française d'Arthroscopie) score for the severity of chondropathy was assigned. At 32 weeks a score was similarly determined for the gross pathologic changes visible on direct examination. In every dog, the score at 32 weeks was higher than that at 16 weeks. The increase between week 16 and week 32 was less marked in the diacerhein (DAR)-treated dogs than in placebo-treated dogs. The p values for the difference between the two treatment groups at week 16 and at week 32 were 0.04 and 0.05, respectively. Reproduced with permission from Smith GN Jr, Myers SL, Brandt KD, *et al.* Diacerhein treatment reduces the severity of osteoarthritis in the canine cruciate-deficiency model of osteoarthritis. *Arthritis Rheum* 1999;42:545–54

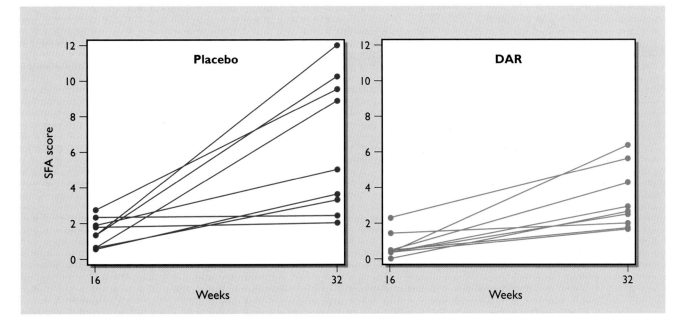

Figure 7 Radioactivity originating from ^{14}C-D-glucosamine. Reproduced with permission from Setnikar I, Palumbo R, Canali S, Zanolo G. Pharmacokinetics of glucosamine in man. *Arzneimittel-Forschung* 1993;43:1109–13

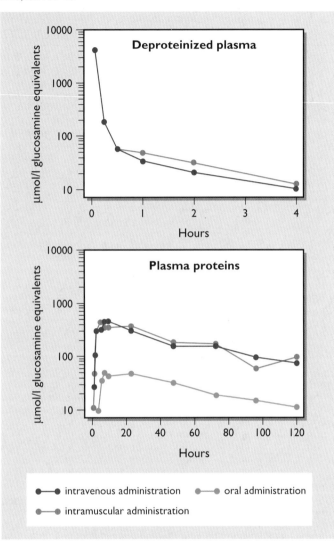

50%, and approximately 7% per year underwent hip arthroplasty (mainly because of rapidly progressive OA), no DMOAD effect of diacerhein was apparent in those with rapid progression. However, among those who completed the study, diacerhein markedly decreased the rate of joint space narrowing in the hip radiograph, mirroring results in the canine OA model and suggesting a DMOAD effect.

Glucosamine sulfate

In a recent preliminary report, mean medial tibiofemoral compartment joint space width was found to decrease 0.24 mm in the placebo group but to increase 0.12 mm in patients treated with glucosamine sulfate over a 3-year interval, suggesting that this treatment had a DMOAD effect. Furthermore, pain scores decreased by some 15% in the glucosamine group but increased 5.5% in the placebo group. However, caution is required in interpreting the changes in joint space width in this study. Narrowing of the medial tibiofemoral compartment joint space in paired standing knee radiographs, as used in this study, may be due to differences in the position of the knee in the two examinations, in the severity of joint pain, in the distance between the knee and the cassette or to other technical factors. Indeed, unless rigorous attention is paid to such detail, the coefficient of variation for joint space width on repeated X-rays of the same knee taken within hours of each other may be as high as 25%.

It is difficult, furthermore, to reconcile the above positive results with the report of Setnikar *et al.*, who were unable to detect radioactivity in deproteinized plasma after oral administration of radiolabeled glucosamine. On the other hand, radioactivity was detectable in serum proteins several hours after ingestion of the radionuclide, suggesting that the lack of free ^{14}C-D-glucosamine in deproteinized plasma was not due to failure to absorb the material, but to first-pass clearance of glucosamine by the liver, where it was subsequently incorporated into plasma proteins (Figure 7). These results suggest that it is unlikely that a significant quantity of glucosamine reaches the joints after oral administration.

Finally, a caveat is required relative to DMOADs in general: as indicated in the chapter on Clinical Features, the cross-sectional correlation between the severity of symptoms and severity of structural damage in an OA joint is poor. A lack of correlation was apparent also in a longitudinal study of 145 patients with knee OA for whom radiographs and clinical data were available at baseline and 3 years later. Although a strong correlation existed between the progression of individual radiographic features of OA (e.g. joint space narrowing, osteophytosis, subchondral sclerosis), no correlation was apparent between the progression of joint pain and disability and the progression of radiographic changes (Table 2).

Bibliography

Altman RD, Howell DS. Disease-modifying osteoarthritis drugs. In Brandt KB, Doherty M, Lohmander LS, eds. *Osteoarthritis*. Oxford: Oxford University Press, 1998:417–28

Amin AR, Attur MG, Thakker GD, *et al.* A novel mechanism of action of tetracyclines: effects on nitric oxide synthases. Proc Natl Acad Sci USA 1996;93:14014–18

Dieppe PA, Cushnaghan J, Shepstone L. The Bristol 'OA500' study: progression of osteoarthritis (OA) over 3 years and the relationship between clinical and radiographic changes in the knee joint. *Osteoarthritis Cartilage* 1997;5:87–97

Doherty M, Jones A. Indomethacin hastens large joint osteoarthritis in humans – how strong is the evidence? *J Rheumatol* 1995;22:2013–16

Ghosh P. The pathobiology of osteoarthritis and the rationale for the use of pentosan poylsulfate for its treatment. *Semin Arthritis Rheum* 1999;28:211–67

Huskisson EC, Berry H, Gishen P, *et al.* Effects of anti-inflammatory drugs on the progression of osteoarthritis of the knee. *J Rheumatol* 1995;22:1941–6

Pavelka K, Gatterová J, Gollerová V, *et al.* A 5 year controlled, double blind study of gylcosaminoglycan polysulphuric acid complex (Rumalon®) as a structure modifying therapy in osteoarthritis of the hip and knee. *Osteoarthritis Cartilage* 2000;in press

Setnikar I, Palumbo R, Canali S, Zanolo G. Pharmacokinetics of glucosamine in man. *Arzneimittel-Forschung* 1993;43:1109–13

Smith GN Jr, Brandt KD, Hasty KA. Procollagenase is reduced to inactive fragments upon activation in the presence of doxycycline. *Ann NY Acad Sci* 1994;732:436–8

Smith GN Jr, Myers SL, Brandt KD, *et al.* Diacerhein treatment reduces the severity of osteoarthritis in the canine cruciate-deficiency model of osteoarthritis. *Arthritis Rheum* 1999;42:545–54

Yu LP Jr, Smith GN Jr, Brandt KD, *et al.* Reduction of the severity of canine osteoarthritis by prophylactic treatment with oral doxycycline. *Arthritis Rheum* 1992;35:1150–9

CHAPTER FIFTEEN

Tidal irrigation of the knee

Figure 1 (a) Joint lavage by tidal irrigation of the knee. The joint space has been entered with a sterile 11-gauge needle after preparation of the skin with antiseptic solution, infiltration of the skin and subcutaneous tissues with local anesthetic down to the joint capsule, and distention of the knee with bupivacaine, a long-acting local anesthetic. (b) The diagram depicts the needle connected to a closed system for delivery of sterile saline and collection of the effluent. The system depicted can be constructed with the supplies used routinely for administration of intravenous fluids. Reproduced with permission from Ike RW. Joint Lavage. In Brandt KD, Doherty M, Lohmander LS, eds. *Osteoarthritis.* London: Oxford University Press, 1998:359–77, © Oxford University Press

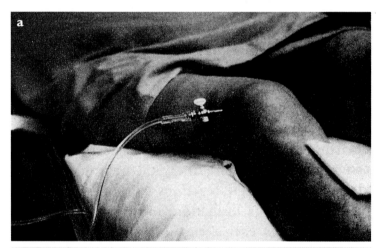

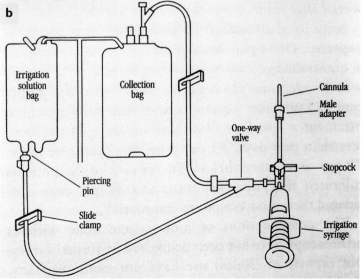

The concept that perfusing an arthritic joint with a large volume of physiologic fluid can sometimes lead to lasting clinical improvement, and thus be worthy of considering as a therapeutic intervention, originated in the writings of the first American arthroscopists. One group describing their initial observations after arthroscopy of the knee noted: "We had the pleasant surprise of seeing a marked improvement of the joint following arthroscopy". One patient who underwent arthroscopy "...had such a good result that he begged us to do the same for the other knee".

The degree to which the lavage associated with the installation of large quantities of saline or Ringer's lactate needed for visualization of intra-articular structures at arthroscopy contributes to the therapeutic result confounds all assessments of arthroscopy as a therapeutic intervention in knee OA. Furthermore, while considerable dexterity and excellent hand–eye coordination are required for proficiency in arthroscopy, joint lavage can be performed by any physician capable of performing an arthrocentesis (Figure 1). Regardless of whether joint lavage is accomplished by a closed needle technique or via arthroscopy, it can be effective in relieving knee pain in certain patients with OA.

At present, therefore, it should be recognized that a number of studies have suggested that tidal irrigation might warrant consideration in any patient with knee OA who might otherwise be considered for arthroscopy. Although several studies have examined the effects of joint lavage in patients with knee OA, most, unfortunately, have not been controlled clinical trials. Because the magnitude of the placebo response to an invasive procedure such as joint lavage is robust and may be sustained, it is difficult to determine to what extent clinical improvement following lavage is due to more than a placebo response. A study designed to address this issue, employing a sham-lavage control group, is currently in progress but the results are not yet available.

The basis for the effectiveness of tidal irrigation in the treatment of knee OA is unclear, but a number of possible contributing factors are listed in Table 1.

Table 1 Possible mechanisms for relief of knee pain in patients with OA after joint lavage

Removal of 'wear particles'

Removal of crystals

Disruption of intra-articular adhesions

Temporary changes:

    Cooling

    Dilution of degradative enzymes

Adapted from Brandt KD. *Diagnosis and Nonsurgical Management of Osteoarthritis*. Caddo OK: Professional Communications, Inc., 1996:1–225

CHAPTER SIXTEEN
Surgical intervention

It is beyond the scope of this monograph to provide a comprehensive discussion of surgery for osteoarthritis. It is important to recognize, however, that surgery plays an important role in the management of this disease. For patients in whom the comprehensive program of medicinal and non-medicinal measures discussed above is ineffective, surgical intervention warrants consideration. Although a variety of surgical procedures, for example soft tissue release, osteotomy and arthrodesis,

may be helpful in individual cases, overwhelmingly, surgical intervention for OA means total joint arthroplasty.

Total hip arthroplasty (THA) (Figure 1) and total knee arthroplasty (TKA) (Figure 2) are, in general, remarkably successful. Pain relief is often striking and the complication rate low. Most subjects who undergo THA or TKA are able to return to essentially full function in activities of daily living. Furthermore, the benefits are typically long

Figure 1 Radiograph of patient who underwent bilateral total hip arthroplasty because of advanced OA, which caused severe hip pain and affected mobility and quality of life

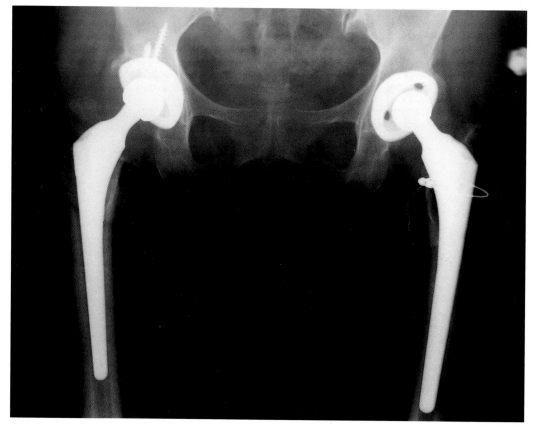

lasting, with the survival rate of the prosthesis now approximately 95% at 10 years and nearly that high at 15 years. If cases of infection are excluded, the success rates for revision of hip and knee arthroplasties which fail at these intervals approximate those for the primary surgery. Given that the patient with severe hip or knee OA is at risk of falling, it is worth noting that the surgical success rate for hip fracture in this individual may be lower than that for total joint arthroplasty.

Physicians often regard orthopaedic intervention for OA as 'radical' and medical management as 'conservative'. However, for the patient with intractable joint discomfort, limited mobility, and a disease which profoundly affects quality of life, continuation of an ineffective medical regimen is, in fact, the 'radical' approach and total joint arthroplasty, the more conservative. Furthermore, excessive delay in total hip or knee replacement, so that patients have poorer physical function and more

pain preoperatively, may result in poorer postoperative improvement, relative to that of patients with higher preoperative function (Tables 1 and 2).

Although OA is a disease whose severity increases with age, the risk of major surgery also increase with age. However, improvements in general medical care and anesthesia technique make arthroplasty a possibility even for the very elderly. With modern surgical techniques and hypotensive epidural anesthesia the mortality of hip arthroplasty was reported only a few years ago to be as low as 0.1%.

Reports of the risk of deep vein thrombosis after arthroplasty have ranged from 10% to 70%, with pulmonary embolism occurring in 1% to 4% of cases. Prophylaxis with, for example, low molecular weight heparin, can reduce the incidence of pulmonary embolism to a negligible level, with few bleeding complications. Similarly excellent results (e.g. 11% deep vein thrombosis and 1% pulmonary

Figure 2 Radiograph of patient who underwent total knee arthroplasty because of severely symptomatic end-stage OA

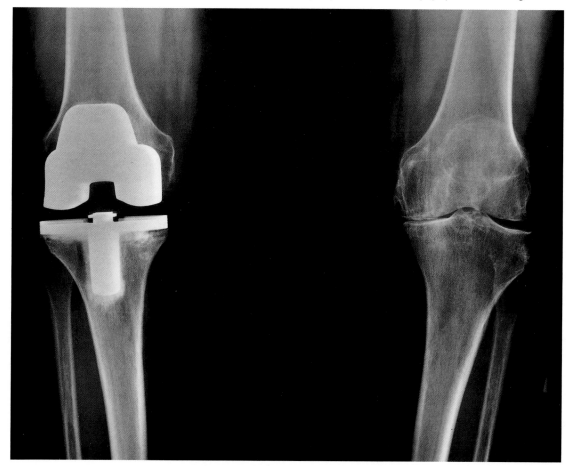

Table I Factors influencing the 'gatekeeper's' decision to refer a patient with knee osteoarthritis to an orthopedic surgeon for consideration of total knee arthroplasty

---

The gatekeeper's ability to make a correct diagnosis

Experience of the gatekeeper

Severity of the disease

Ability of the gatekeeper to assess disease severity

Attitude of the gatekeeper toward orthopaedic surgery, in general,

and TKA, in particular

Relationship of the gatekeeper to local orthopaedic surgeons

Access to orthopaedic surgery

Access to alternatives, such as physical therapy

Presence of referral guidelines

Cost

From Dieppe P, Basler H-D, Chard J, et al. Knee replacement surgery for osteoarthritis: effectiveness, practice variation, indications and possible determinants of utilization. *Rheumatology* 1999;38:73–83

embolism) may be achieved with hypotensive epidural anesthesia and aspirin therapy.

Late local complications of arthroplasty include deep infection, loosening, osteolysis, periprosthetic fractures, implant wear and breakage. Wear is unlikely to cause problems during the first ten years after surgery, but can result in instability and dislocation of the joint. Some 80% of all THA revisions are performed because of loosening, the risk of which is approximately 10% at 10 years and is greater in men and younger patients than in women and older patients (Figure 3). Osteolysis triggered by wear particles can reduce the amount of bone stock needed for subsequent revision.

The overall infection rate after THA is less than 1%. In patients with medical contraindications to surgery, antibiotics alone may slow down the destructive process. However, in most cases, deep infection is best treated by removal of the implant and other foreign material and debridement of the infected tissue, with prolonged antibiotic therapy based on the results of cultures.

Table 2 Physical function and pain 6 months after total hip replacement in patients who had high or low function at baseline*

Outcome measure	High function at baseline		Low function at baseline		Difference high – low	
	Mean ± SD	95% CI	Mean ± SD	95% CI	Mean	95% CI
SF-36 physical function						
Baseline	35.6 ± 23.5		16.7 ± 16.7		19.0	11.5, 26.4
6 months	68.0 ± 23.0		51.5 ± 26.6		16.4	7.3, 25.5
Difference						
(6 months – baseline)	32.5	26.3, 38.8	35.0	28.1, 42.0	–2.5	–11.8, 6.8
WOMAC pain						
Baseline	8.5 ± 3.3		12.2 ± 3.5		–3.7	–4.9, –2,4
6 months	1.9 ± 2.2		3.7 ± 3.8		–1.9	–3.0, –0.7
Difference						
(6 months – baseline)	–6.6	–7.5, –5.6	–8.3	–9.5, –7.2	1.8	0.3, 3.3
WOMAC function						
Baseline	27.4 ± 9.2		47.5 ± 6.3		–20.1	–22.9, –17.2
6 months	10.8 ± 8.3		16.7 ± 11.9		–5.9	–9.7, –2.1
Difference						
(6 months – baseline)	–16.6	–19.3, –14.0	–30.2	–33.3, –27.2	13.6	9.6, 17.5

*The Western Ontario and McMaster Universities Osteoarthritis Index (WOMAC) subscale scores are a summation of the subscale itemized scores. A value of 'zero' was assigned if 'none' was the answer reported, and a value of '4' if extreme' was reported. Therefore, the range for WOMAC pain is 0–20 and for WOMAC function, 0–68. For the Short Form 36 (SF-36), a higher score represents better function; for WOMAC, a higher score represents worse limitation. 95% CI, 95% confidence interval. Reproduced with permission from Fortin PR, Clarke AE, Joseph L, et al. Outcomes of total hip and knee replacement. Preoperative functional status predicts outcomes at six months after surgery. *Arthritis Rheum* 1999;42:1722–8

Figure 3 Survival rates, in relation to age of patient at the time of surgery, for hip arthroplasties performed in Sweden from 1978 to 1990. From Malchau H, Herberts P, Ahnfelt L. Prognosis of total hip replacement in Sweden: follow-up of operations performed in 1978–1990. *Acta Orthop Scand* 1993;64:497–506

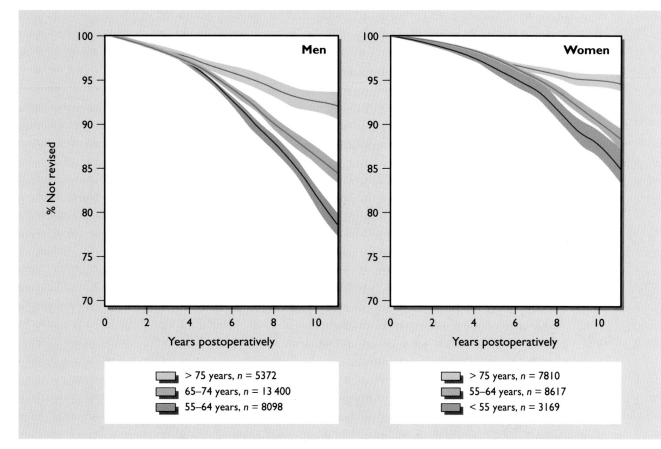

Knutson has succinctly reviewed the local complications after TKA. Based on an analysis of the Swedish knee arthroplasty registry, some 6% of revisions after TKA are performed for patellar problems, 7% for instability and 15% for other mechanical reasons. Loosening is the indication underlying approximately half of all revisions after TKA. However, the cumulative risk for revision 10 years after surgery is now as low as 3%. The risk is twice as great with unicondylar implants as with total knee implants. The cumulative risk of revision for deep infection after TKA is less than 1% at 10 years.

Several studies have confirmed that TKA reduces knee pain and improves function and quality of life in patients with knee OA and it is the recommended treatment for severe knee OA when medical therapy has been unsuccessful. On the other hand, controlled trials of TKA are scarce and no trials have been published which compare TKA with any other intervention. In most published studies, survival of the prosthesis is the primary (and often only) outcome measure, rather than patient-oriented outcomes. There are no evidence-based indications for TKA in patients with knee OA. The incidence rate for joint arthroplasty varies widely among countries and even among geographic regions within the same country. For example, among individuals over the age of 65 years, approximately 0.5–0.7 per 10 000 population TKAs are performed in the UK and Canada, but more than 2 per 1000 in the United States. It is widely considered that severe daily pain associated with loss of joint space width on the knee radiograph are the chief indications for TKA, whereas co-morbid conditions and technical difficulties are reasons for not performing the procedure.

It is unclear which patients will benefit most from the procedure. It has been suggested that TKA is under-utilized. Dieppe *et al.* have recently published a thoughtful analysis of why some individuals, but not others, with knee OA seek medical attention and the factors that determine whether such individuals are referred to an orthopaedic surgeon. Patients who are obese are often told that surgery cannot be performed until they lose weight (which they find difficult to accomplish). However, there is no evidence that obesity results in a poorer outcome. A particular problem which warrants consideration is that people who attribute their symptoms to aging are more likely to consider that nothing can be done to help and less likely, therefore, to seek medical attention. Indeed, joint pain in the elderly may be ignored because it is thought of as a normal consequence of aging.

Finally, it should be noted that a number of investigative surgical procedures, such as autologous chondrocyte transplantation, use of mesenchymal stem cells, and autologous osteochondral plugs (mosaicplasty) are being evaluated for their utility in the repair of isolated chondral defects, such as those caused by traumatic injury. None of these procedures, however, is currently indicated for the treatment of OA. Excellent reviews of the current status of research on regeneration of articular cartilage and articular cartilage transplantation have been published recently.

Bibliography

Brittberg M, Nilsson A, Lindahl A, *et al.* Rabbit articular cartilage defects treated with autologous cultured chondrocytes. *Clin Orthop Rel Res* 1996;362:270–83

Buckwalter JA, Mankin HJ. Articular cartilage repair and transplantation. *Arthritis Rheum* 1998;41:1331–42

Dieppe P, Basler H-D, Chard J, *et al.* Knee replacement surgery for osteoarthritis: effectiveness, practice variations, indications and possible determinants of utilization. *Rheumatology* 1999;38:73–83

Freund DA, Dittus RS. Assessing and improving outcomes: total knee replacement. Final report of the patient outcomes research team (PORT). Washington, AHCPR Pub. No. 97- N015, 1997

Knutson K. Arthroplasty and its complications. In Brandt KD, Doherty M, Lohmander LS, eds. *Osteoarthritis.* Oxford: Oxford University Press, 1998:388–402

O'Driscoll SW. Current Concepts Review: The healing and regeneration of articular cartilage. *J Bone Joint Surg* 1998;80A:1795–812

Wakitani S, Goto T, Pineda SJ, *et al.* Mesenchymal cell-based repair of large, full-thickness defects of articular cartilage. *J Bone Joint Surg Am* 1994;76A:579–92

Wright JG, Coyte P, Hawker G, *et al.* Variation in orthopaedic surgeons' perceptions of the indications for and outcomes of knee replacement. *Can Med Assoc J* 1995;152:687–97

INDEX

Entries in **bold** indicate figures.